Praise for *No Shame*

• • • •

"Dr. Lea Lis' brilliant book explains that when parents own their sexual story, it allows them to pass down intergenerational wisdom—not trauma. *No Shame* addresses the prevalent shame and fear around sexuality, and Dr. Lis' fresh approach to communication with children on those awkward topics gives parents the tools they need to help their kids develop body positivity, self-esteem, and healthy romantic relationships."

Dr. Shefali Tsabary, bestselling author of *The Conscious Parent*

"Dr. Lea Lis provides parents with a field manual of evidence-based practices to help us discuss the dos and don'ts of relationships, intimacy, and sex with our kids. Drawing on her decades of work in the trenches as a clinician and her own experiences as a parent, the Shameless Psychiatrist has given us a treasure trove of tools and techniques that you will come back to again and again."

Jess P. Shatkin, MD, MPH, author of *Born to Be Wild,* professor at NYU Grossman School of Medicine, and host of *About Our Kids*

"I wish I'd had a book like this that brought up vocabulary and ways to talk to your kids about self-confidence, boundaries, and healthy relationships when I was raising my kids."

Susan Sarandon, actor and activist

"Dr. Lea Lis has written *the* modern guide on talking to kids about sex. Part parent, part sex therapist, and part coach, Dr. Lis addresses countless topics parents often shy away from simply because they're uncomfortable; her guidance is both sound and sage, backed by science and written with tact and grace. *No Shame* helps us separate fact from fiction in healthy child sexual development."

Goali Saedi Bocci, PhD, licensed clinical psychologist and author of *The Millennial Mental Health Toolbox*

"Dr. Lea Lis offers parents many practical insights on when, why, and how to engage in open and developmentally appropriate conversations about sexuality. If the thought of talking with your child about sex makes you uncomfortable, this book is for you."

William C. Wood, MD, clinical assistant professor of psychiatry at Weill Cornell Medicine

"The Shameless Psychiatrist has written a thoughtful book about ways families can better communicate and engage. *No Shame* is very clear, organized, and practical; parents will use it over and over again as a reference."

Scott M. Palyo, MD, child and adolescent psychiatrist and assistant clinical professor at New York Medical College

"Dr. Lea Lis' recommendations are outstanding. Her advice is based on the latest scientific research, as well as being rooted in her lengthy experience working with parents and children to develop healthy communication and relationships. Everyone can benefit from her insights."

Dr. Katherine Frank, cultural anthropologist, sex researcher, writer, and life/sex/wellness coach

"As a clinical researcher who works with children with autism spectrum disorder, I think Dr. Lea Lis has done an excellent job in addressing sexual education for and sexuality in teenagers who struggle with basic romantic relationships. *No Shame* will be very useful for parents in helping their children who are on the spectrum."

Dr. Alex Kolevzon, child and adolescent psychiatrist and professor of psychiatry and pediatrics at the Icahn School of Medicine at Mount Sinai

"If you don't start the dialogue with your kids about sex, who or what will you leave it to? Snapchat? The dark web? The Shameless Psychiatrist covers all the bases in this hands-on guide that really delivers. Thought-provoking, insightful, and timely, this book just might become your new parenting bible!"

Dr. Melissa Angiel, psychologist

"Dr. Lea Lis is changing the way we talk about sex with our children. This is book is educational, connecting, and, most importantly, an extreme asset for all parents."

Abbey Williams, MSW, LSW, host of *Mimosas with Moms*

"Refreshingly contemporary, *No Shame* addresses how parents can help kids navigate conflicts and the challenges of growing up in the world of #MeToo and social media."

Cristina Cuomo, founder and editor of *The Purist*

No Shame

No Shame

Real Talk with Your Kids about Sex, Self-Confidence, and Healthy Relationships

Dr. Lea Lis

The Shameless Psychiatrist

PAGE TWO BOOKS

THIS BOOK IS DEDICATED to the people of New York. They provided me with the experiences I needed to write it and the motivation I needed to become a doctor. I was at Ground Zero as an intern at Saint Vincent's Hospital in 2001. The OR had a perfect view of downtown. Someone pointed to a fire in the Twin Towers and then we all watched as the second plane hit. With fire trucks screaming down 7th Avenue, we did not realize that many of the firemen in those trucks would not make it back. Shards were flying from the sky while I watched thousands of people wander up from downtown, all white as ghosts. These were the days of camaraderie when everyone said hello to one another—such pure love from strangers. I am now back, during the COVID-19 pandemic, as a volunteer; many doctors have become infected and some have even died. It takes me right back to my feeling—scared but grateful—for all that New York has given me. When this book is published, I hope there will be an end to this crisis for the people of New York.

Contents

1

An Introduction to Shameless Psychiatry

The what, why, & how of positive parenting
• • • •

Education is not permission

Don't you want your children to be autonomous, sexually fulfilled adults? Don't you want your children to have successful and loving intimate relationships? Helping them to do so means being sex-positive. The phrase "sex-positive" in association with parenting is sometimes misunderstood as taking a permissive or "anything goes" approach to sexuality... No, that's simply not the case! It's not permissive parenting; it's an extension of overall positive parenting. It also means teaching them how to communicate, how to live without shame, teaching them to love their bodies, how to be vulnerable. You need to nurture your child's sexual development, through adolescence and into adulthood, by educating them to understand not only the pleasures *and* the dangers of sexual activity, but also how sexual activity can enhance their relationships, and help foster intimacy. This book is not just about sexual education; it is about the roles that sex and sexuality play in the healthy development of intimate relationships.

Communication can be so hard... but you gotta do it!

Parents, here's the most important thing to remember: developing a parent-child relationship based on mutual trust, respect, and openness sets the stage for your child to build self-esteem and develop

3

healthy relationships throughout their life. Good communication allows you to impart your values to your child and helps them to in turn navigate an increasingly complicated world. Your communication patterns with your child should start when they are very young and will be replicated in their future relationships, so whatever your patterns are early on... that's what your child will likely continue with into their adult life. Start setting a good example now. And if, after reading this book, you feel you've made mistakes in the past, now is the time to correct them.

Here are some facts to back all this up:

- Parent-adolescent communication plays a protective role in adolescent sexual behavior, leading to later sexual initiation, more consistent condom use, and less risky behavior.

- Teens who have regular conversations with their parents about sex also report having closer relationships with them overall.

- A powerful study of the link between parent-adolescent communication and safer sex practices among youth examined 30 years of data from more than 25,000 adolescents. Researchers found parent-adolescent sexual communication influenced safer sex behavior, such as the use of contraceptives and condoms.

- Communication with parents about sexual matters was also associated with increased communication with dating partners.

Unfortunately, research also shows that too few adolescents talk with *anyone* about sexual topics—neither parents, friends, nor dating partners—and that attempts at such conversations fail when sex is defined only as a source of disease or the possibility of conversation is silenced through authoritative proscription of having sex at all. Don't let your child be the one left in the dark.

So, start those talks early on and keep them going!

Do you want to be the kind of parent who shuts down sex discussions, leaving it up to your child's school, their friends, and pornography to dictate the messages they learn? No way! You know you have a unique opportunity to do better than the way you may have been raised, and that's why you've come to this book. You have the opportunity to send the kind of messages that impart your values and your truth.

Sex is not something that should only be talked about once, or only in times of crisis

What is the right age to begin to talk to your child about sex? As soon as they can speak! Rather than being compressed into a single monologue, as in a one-off "Talk," something that generations who came of age in the 1950s, '60s, '70s, and '80s experienced, a sex-positive education should begin at birth and continue throughout a child's life, with developmentally appropriate explanations and discussions.

Unfortunately, even parents who communicate effectively with their children in almost every other situation become tongue-tied or nervous when it comes to sex. Further, given children's inevitable exposure to a sex-saturated media, and to a host of contemporary social debates about gender and sexuality, such discussions need to happen not only earlier but with greater frequency, and have become more challenging for parents.

Just to reiterate this important point: As a parent, you may fail to address issues around sex, gender, reproduction, and identity during your children's earlier years because you worry about seeming overly permissive or attracting undue attention to the subject of sex. Or, you may simply not know how or when to start. Some parents may also worry that kids will be tempted to experiment if they acquire any bit of sexual knowledge. But this logic is backwards: warning your kids about a cliff doesn't necessarily make them want to jump off!

Many parents thus leave the important job of sex education to the schools, but sex education is rarely taught early enough or well enough in the classroom. Most contemporary sexual issues are not addressed in public school sex education programs, and schools vary in terms of the content they offer. By middle school, vast differences in knowledge develop among peers due to their parents' political, religious, and other beliefs—not to mention their fears. Don't leave this important job to the schools. Take the matter into your own hands. I am here to help you do so with competence and ease.

Parent Public Service Announcement!

So, with all that being said, I have a Parent Public Service Announcement: *knowledge protects children at each phase of their development.*

Here are some recent statistics:

- About 1 in 10 children will be sexually abused before their 18th birthday.

- About 1 in 7 girls and 1 in 25 boys will be sexually abused before they turn 18.

- 44 percent of rapes with penetration occur to children under age 18.

- Victims younger than 12 account for 15 percent of those raped, and another 29 percent of rape victims are between 12 and 17.

Children are most vulnerable to sexual abuse and assault at ages when many parents have not yet even broached the subject of sex.

Starting a child's sex education early has a protective effect. Very young children who do not know the proper words for their genitals, for example, are at risk for sexual victimization because they cannot easily provide a description if something happens to them. Older children who have developed shame around their sexuality may decide to keep their victimization secret rather than share details with a trusted adult like you. Adolescents and older teenagers often turn to their friends–and, increasingly, the Internet–for advice and information rather than their parents... and we know how reliable the Internet is for information.

Rapidly changing world

Children today are growing up in a rapidly changing world. As a parent, you may be single, divorced, cohabiting, or remarried. The children that you currently have may be the result of previous partnerships, adoption, or a variety of reproductive technologies. You may be in a same-sex partnership, multiple partnerships, or outside-the-box co-parenting arrangements, which are becoming more prevalent and more visible. New understandings of sex and gender, along with a range of alternative identities, have ushered in even more possibilities for relationships and families.

As a parent, you hope to prepare your child to lead a successful, meaningful, and satisfied life, even though you may feel uncertainty about what the future looks like. The hopes and fears of parents drive an expanding literary offering on the subject of parenting: parenting after divorce, stepparenting, single parenting, same-sex parenting, parenting the adopted child, parenting the LGBTQ+ child, and so on. To further complicate matters, many family arrangements are not necessarily mutually exclusive. For example, two lesbians might form a "blended" family: raising one child conceived in a prior opposite-sex union and one child they adopted together. Identities are not mutually exclusive either: a parent might be single, nonmonogamous, *and* bisexual. And, regardless of your own family arrangement, all parents and children will undoubtedly encounter gender, sexual, and relationship diversity.

Children thrive in loving and respectful environments... period.

Whether such social changes are positive or negative, for society or for individuals, is not up for debate in this book. My goal in *No Shame: Real Talk with Your Kids about Sex, Self-Confidence, and Healthy Relationships* is to help parents in any type of family arrangement raise strong, secure, and resilient children who become strong, secure, and resilient adults—an aspiration that resonates across the lines of identity and sexuality. After spending more than a decade as a psychiatrist working with parents and children in almost every imaginable type of family, I believe that children thrive in loving and respectful environments. It's that simple—and that complicated.

So now let's talk about the how-to

My approach to the nuts and bolts of sex education is developmentally appropriate and can be adapted to work with the beliefs and values of your family. Ever since Jean Piaget, a famous psychologist, began to study the development of children, psychologists and psychiatrists have studied and refined our understanding of human cognitive development. What was once thought of as a hierarchy of discrete, identifiable developmental "stages" is now viewed as a continuum; human maturation from infancy to adulthood is understood as a dynamic process rather than a one-time achievement. Still, the process of learning how to think, remember, and interact with others is similar enough across time and place to serve as a map, even if some of the territory is uncharted.

Drawing on insights from cognitive psychology, *No Shame* presents parents with

- time-tested strategies for tackling common (as well as uncommon) problems, concerns, and situations associated with each developmental stage;

- emotional regulation techniques, such as mindfulness, that can be taught at each stage;

- resources for further reading; and

- discussion topics for parents and older children.

These techniques can be adapted and practiced over time by you and your child to enhance communication, strengthen relationships, regulate emotions, and build self-esteem.

Communicate in the NOW

Parents, here's another important reality to keep in mind: Some of our knowledge about sexuality remains stable over time. But there will always be new research, an ever-changing social context, and the fact that beliefs about sex are always understood within the framework of our current values, which are also ever-changing. This means that we parents periodically need to revisit what we have learned. Our children may also need to tackle issues that never even occurred to us. For example, when we were young gay marriage was illegal and almost a taboo topic. Then we watched it come to the political forefront as a hot-button issue in the last couple of decades. Now, for our youngest round of children, gay marriage seems like a total non-issue, and you may be discovering their attention is on trans rights and freedom from the social construct of gender.

This book thus also prepares you to handle questions and concerns that fall outside a basic sex education but are increasingly part of growing up today: sexual identities, the composition of contemporary families, the changing world of dating, the accessibility of pornography, sex in the media, the pressures of social media on youth, and other dizzying topics. I am seeing an uptick in confusion about gender identity and sexual orientation in my practice. This leaves many teens stressed about their identity in this ever-changing societal dynamic, and they are getting very little guidance from mentors and parents, who are often just as confused themselves.

In addition, teenagers today are facing a crisis of intimacy in their relationships. Boys are pushed to have no-strings-attached sex from early on... as early as their first sexual encounters. Girls are having sex to gain attention rather than for pleasure or intimacy, and are pushed from young ages to present themselves in a sexualized manner. Sexual liberation can sometimes become confused with a lack of personal boundaries or self-respect.

Parents, you need to address pleasure as a main element in sex ed! Moms, can you imagine the impact it would have had on your own empowerment if your parents had actually told you that what matters during sex is *your* pleasure? I mean, wow, what a revolutionary concept! We'll be diving into this idea of including the importance of pleasure in your sex ed communications later in this book.

Here's another big one: the line between consent and coercion is often debated in the media—think of the #MeToo movement—but remains fuzzy for adolescents attempting to navigate their relationships. When you were in eighth grade, you probably never had to figure out how to handle requests for naked selfies over Snapchat. You may never have processed a breakup that happened over text message. But that is all the more reason to communicate with your child about the unique challenges they are confronting.

You are about to get some awesome therapy tips

Parents, this book is not just aiming to give you advice about sexual education. This book is so much more! I am a practical therapist who uses cutting-edge therapeutic tools to make my patients well. I use these same tools to give great advice about raising a sex-positive child. I am giving you the best of all the little pearls from the evidence-based therapy I use in my medical practice. Take these pearls as a huge value-add in your parenting toolbox. I have seen the common problems faced by children, and I will teach you what you need to know both with tips and with patient stories to illuminate the important points. Please be advised these are all fictionalized accounts of patient experiences I have had over the years; names and identifying information have been changed to protect patients' privacy, which I hold sacred.

Who is the Shameless Psychiatrist?

So, here is my origin story. By age 15, I already knew I wanted to be a child psychiatrist. My aunt Marie, to whom I was very close, was a psychiatric social worker. She developed a unique style for treating severely mentally ill patients, such as those with schizophrenia. Rather than just recording a patient's responses to her questions, Marie took an authoritative role and gave them instructions to follow. Her commanding presence, along with her integrative approach to treatment and rehabilitation, made for many successful cases in the facilities where she worked. I didn't know at the time the fundamental influence her style of therapy would have on my own practice later on.

When I was 15, Marie signed me up as a volunteer and found ways to take me into the locked wards to help her interview. This was unheard of at the time, and it probably would never be allowed today. I was the only sophomore at Manhasset Secondary School ever to work on a locked psychiatric ward. It was a profoundly life-changing experience, one that set me apart from my friends. Like other kids, I worried about where I would sit at lunch and if I would be invited to the cool parties, but at the same time I also worried that a patient I was working with might have an aggressive outburst that morning. Part of me cared about what I was planning to wear to the next dance, but another part thought that dances were frivolous compared with caring for people who were mentally ill. My classmates had no idea what I did after school and on weekends, and I wouldn't have known how to begin to explain it to them.

At a young age, I discovered that I had an intense empathy with others. I have always been the person everyone comes to with their problems and for my advice. Although it was shocking for me to work with those patients who were so severely ill, it also set me on a course to study psychology and to start thinking about what we—as humans, as members of a certain culture, and as individuals—do and do not want to talk about. I became fascinated with the human mind. I logged many hours talking with patients and the professionals who cared for them.

Discovering my calling and choosing my career so young meant that I was able to focus my energy and time on taking the most direct path to my goal: high school, undergraduate college, medical school, internship, and eventually building a private practice. I also had that "ten thousand hours" of experience early on, which, coupled with my innate understanding, allowed me to become an expert. I can diagnose many patients after the first sentence they utter just by the way they walk into my office, their body language, and their initial facial expressions.

It was also as a teenager that I became aware that people who did not conform to mainstream ideals of gender, sexuality, or relationship style were stigmatized and ostracized. My great-uncle Frank brought his "special friend" Bob with him to family gatherings. It took me years to realize that he was gay. They were both accepted as members of the family, although none of us talked about the true nature of their relationship. To Frank and Bob, adopting a child would have been unthinkable, even if it had been their dream to marry or have a family together.

Now, I am familiar with research showing that marriage and family can provide health benefits and social support networks that are important across sexual orientations or preferences. But even back then, the fact that people would be barred from fulfilling such dreams seemed unfair to me, and even destructive.

It was while I was weighing the unfairness of how society treats us based on our sexuality that I met an HIV patient named Matthew. I was 17 and volunteering on a locked ward at Hillside Hospital, and Matthew was only two years older than me, but dying of diseases related to HIV. Despite being so painfully thin, his body riddled with sores, he smiled when I entered the room. He also had dementia. When he was lucid, he sometimes told me stories about his lovers. My friendship with Matthew left an indelible impression on me, because what he was going through seemed so cruel. He would never travel or fall in love again. He wouldn't even celebrate his 21st birthday. And because AIDS was still thought of as a "gay disease" then in the US, he was blamed for his own misfortune.

This experience stuck with me. I began studying psychology and neuroscience at Dartmouth College, and continued to work at Hillside as a researcher. In 1999, I entered medical school at St. Vincent's in New York City. At the height of the AIDS panic, many hospitals were turning away homosexual men. St. Vincent's is a Catholic hospital and, remarkably, opened its doors to a community that was being hit hard by an epidemic that was still little understood. For several years I worked on the St. Vincent's wards dedicated to treating these patients. Later, I also worked in an HIV clinic where patients were suffering from mental illnesses that had been triggered by the disease. These ailments included cognitive impairments and depression.

The sense of loss experienced by these men overwhelmed me. Society prevented men with same-sex partners from loving each other openly, marrying, and raising children together. Sometimes their own families had deserted them out of shame or fear. And now a disease was destroying the only social ties they had left, killing their lovers, partners, and friends.

By 2003, when I started my residency at New York University School of Medicine, HIV was better understood and on its way to being controlled—at least among some groups. Gay and lesbian communities were slowly regrouping, with an enhanced emphasis on creating cho-sen "families." Although progress was uneven, gay men and lesbians were increasingly living openly with their partners, sometimes with children. Researchers, health professionals, and politicians raised concerns that single or gay fathers would not make good parents because they were not as nurturing as women, or that alternative fam-ily arrangements would generate instability because partners could not be married. Some people even suggested that children in nontra-ditional families would be exposed to inappropriate sexual scenarios in addition to debilitating social stigma.

How I learned the secret sauce for raising healthy children

As a child psychiatrist, I knew that good parenting requires love, support, and setting boundaries for the child. Parents who were great role models and mentors raised successful children. Being a good role model and mentor was more important than whether the parents worked outside the home or baked homemade cookies every day.

When I began working with the children of gay parents, I real-ized that the basic ingredients of good parenting were the same in those homes as well. Nontraditional family structures posed some unique challenges, but overall, children traveled similar developmen-tal routes regardless of the sexual orientation of their parents.

For the lesbians I saw in my practice, parenting was intentional rather than accidental. Pregnancy wasn't–*couldn't be*–the result of a drunken night. They attended to details that would be taken for granted by straight parents. Before gay marriage was legal, for example, same-sex partners worked out legal parenting agreements in addition to wills and other documents to protect their children. Lesbians sought out male role models for their kids, as they knew that opposite-sex attachments and interactions would be important. They consulted with me even though I often thought they did not really need my advice–their children were well-cared-for and well-adjusted. When they realized that I was accepting of their sexuality, they referred other clients to me. After I started my practice, Mindful Kid, in 2008 in the Hamptons, my practice grew and I knew I was gaining the experience I needed to write this book.

During this time, gay men were also increasingly becoming parents through surrogacy and adoption. Although I found that the lack of a "mom" could make parenting a bit more complicated for these families, the difficulties could be addressed. The gay male couples that I worked with, for example, did not always realize that one of them might need to take time off work during the early months of their child's life. They wanted to rely on a baby nurse to do this work, even though research shows that developing a stable early attachment with a primary caregiver is extremely important for a child's development. I would counsel them on choosing roles for the child's first few months, whether that of the caregiver, who takes a lengthy paternity leave of at least three months, or that of the breadwinner, who provides the financial and other support during that period. These roles are usually gendered in heterosexual families, although they do not need to be. Once the men realized they couldn't take the value of such early "mothering" lightly, they stepped up to the challenge.

I could say the same applies to modern-minded heterosexual couples where both members are breadwinners. I am finding that more and more fathers are deciding to take a step back from their career to be the primary caregiver, as their partner may have either a more lucrative career or a higher societal impact career. *And* the father may be more suited to the nurturing role. See the documentary about Ruth Bader Ginsberg and her husband, who supported her every step of the way with both parenting and behind-the-scenes advocacy work in the service of her rise to the US Supreme Court. Not only did RBG live an untraditional life (especially during the 1970s!), but she stressed the need for all parents to have their rights protected, regardless of gender, in her earliest Supreme Court cases.

My permanent shift away from gender bias

People like RBG have shown us that anyone can take either a traditionally masculine or a traditionally feminine role when it comes to parenting. Debates raged in the media, and sometimes the courts, over whether gay and lesbian parents could be "good parents." But every day in my practice, I saw real-life examples of conscientious, loving, effective parenting by same-sex couples. And as the scientists began to weigh in with research on the question, it became clear that parenting was not the privileged domain of heterosexuals. Same-sex partners could do just as good a job as opposite-sex partners, by some measures even better. They did, however, face some unique issues as well. As I began systematically thinking about how best to help non-traditional families move through the different phases of child rearing, the initial ideas for this book began taking shape.

In 2009, while pregnant with my first daughter, I had another significant experience. I attended the Burning Man festival—an annual gathering of hippies, artists, and cultural visionaries that takes place in the desert near Reno, Nevada. For one week, Black Rock City becomes a temporary "home" for thousands of people experimenting with the concept of community. Burning Man is based on the principles of cooperation, self-reliance, self-expression, and "radical inclusion." I found the concept of radical inclusion to be compelling. All ages are welcome at the festival. Kidsville is an area of the city where parents and their children set up a kibbutz-like camp.

Similarly, all sexualities are welcome at the festival. Black Rock City ideas of radical expression mean that all forms of sexual expression are accepted; for example, cross-dressing is accepted and even encouraged. This open-mindedness of "burners" was fascinating to me. I was flabbergasted by the theme on Tuesday at Burning Man, called Tutu Tuesday. Thousands of men, women, and children dressed in all-color tutus as a celebration of the whimsical. Even heteronormative men loved wearing tutus and playing around with their sexual expression in a place where they knew they would be accepted. The people I met there tended to be accepting of differences in practice and belief. As long as no one was being hurt, there was no reason to object to how others wanted to live their lives, whether for that one week or throughout the rest of the year. The notion is simple yet somehow transformative in its contrast to our default real world.

Through my networks at Burning Man, I met people who had formed multi-parent households—communities of lovers and ex-lovers who took an interest in raising children together. Some households were composed of parents who had moved on sexually but chose to remain intact as co-parents and friends. Other households were made up of multiple romantic and sexual partners. The parents might identify as straight, gay, lesbian, transgender, polyamorous—or none of these things. Sometimes in nontraditional families, children were getting *more* attention, not less. They had more people to turn to for social support or mentoring. They were receiving love from multiple parental figures... and they were *thriving*.

The traditional psychological positions on parenting that I was exposed to during my training had tended to be conservative, promoting the nuclear family as necessary for the development of a healthy, mature child. But once again, in real life, I was seeing that diversity in family structure did not necessarily lead to psychopathology or other negative outcomes. I brought these observations and experiences back into my practice, paying even closer attention to how child-rearing challenges could be both universal (i.e., creating a safe, supportive environment for early learning and navigating the stormy emotional waters of adolescence) and more specific (as when same-sex parents anticipate that their children will experience stigma and bullying).

Why listen to the "Shame Less!" Psychiatrist?

I am a double board-certified adult and child psychiatrist trained at NY Medical College and NYU. I am active in the American Psychiatric Association, having served as a member of their National Ethics Committee and a member of the Board of Trustees. I have presented numerous symposia and workshops at the APA annual meetings, as well as at the meetings of the Institute of Psychiatric Services. My publications have appeared in the *Journal of Psychiatric Practice* and *Academic Psychiatry*, and I continue to conduct research in my field.

I am a mouthpiece in the mainstream media, having appeared as an expert on parenting on ABC, CBS, NBC, and other news outlets;

in newspapers (*Chicago Tribune, Washington Post*); in niche publications (*Modern Beach Luxury, Psychiatric News*); in online articles; and in blogs.

During my training and residency at St. Vincent's Hospital in New York and New York University, as well as in my ongoing private psychiatric practice, Mindful Kid, I have developed expertise in working with modern families, from children of multiracial adoption to those with parents identifying as gay, lesbian, or transgender. I have so many powerful stories to share of patients with problems that I would like to share. I'm always looking for opportunities to bring my clinical experience to a broader audience, offering nuts-and-bolts strategies for tackling common (and uncommon) problems, concerns, and situations arising around sexuality at each developmental stage.

My goal is to give you critically important information in a humorous and compelling way about everyone's favorite topic: sex! This will be a fun read. ☺ With this book, I will help you as you strive to do what is right for your children by merging the knowledge I obtained in my conventional training as a psychiatrist with the openness to diversity that I have gained through my personal relationships and experiences.

The main insights I hope to impart to you are these:

- Anyone can be a good parent.

- Healthy relationships are critical.

- Owning your own sexual story will help you have better relationships and be a better parent.

Mind hacking
· · · ·

This book will guide you in this communication journey with your child, and help you navigate our rapidly changing world. In addition to an emphasis on overall positive—and specifically sex-positive—parenting from birth through adolescence and early adulthood, *No Shame* presents techniques and strategies drawn from two prominent behavioral therapies—cognitive behavioral therapy (CBT) and dialectical behavior therapy (DBT)—to teach you (the parent) and your child to improve your emotional states and your interactions with each other.

What is a "thought hole"? It's a cycle of negative thinking or a skewed perception that you get caught in. The reason I'm bringing up these thought hole disruptor therapies is that they can give you the tools to untangle narratives that you choose to recognize as your own story. Your sexual story—a combination of all your experiences, fears, pleasures, and memories rolled up into a ball—is the narrative you bring to the table when you speak to your children about sex. And it should be a positive one if you want to pass down wisdom rather than trauma. You, parents, can use these therapies to help reframe your sexual story into something that enables you to be a better role model for your kids. Use these disruptors to help yourself develop a better interpersonal relationship with them overall and foster a better communication system about sex. Strong communication about sex is necessary to create children who become adults with happy, healthy, body-positive, shame-free sex lives.

Mind Hack Level 1: CBT is a thought hole disruptor

Perception is reality. When one person walks down a street, they see the ice cream store and the flower boxes, while another person sees graffiti and litter. And yet they are walking down the same street.

We are taking millions of morsels of information into our sensory system every second. What we tune ourselves into can make the difference between a happy, well-adjusted human and a miserable, low-confidence human. Cognitive distortions, or thought holes, are like images that have been filtered through a fun-house mirror— distorted, odd-looking, unreal. It is by means of cognitive distortions that you may come to certain troubling conclusions, such as "He gave me a look, so he must hate me" or "Why does she look so much better than me in the same pants?" This distortion of reality makes us feel depressed, contributes to self-esteem issues, and frankly leads us believe we are not sexy, therefore taking away from our enjoyment of life and, for the purpose of this book, our enjoyment of sex!

So here's the deal with CBT: Emotions can't be changed directly. If someone tells you to be happy, are you happy? Um, no. But you *can* change your behaviors (for example, exercise can make you feel better) and your thoughts ("Maybe they *do* want me to come to the party!"). And both of those changes can bring about a change in your emotions. CBT is a type of therapy that focuses on the development of personal coping strategies that aim to solve current problems and change unhelpful patterns in thoughts or behaviors (thought holes).

CBT has proven valuable for troubled families marked by conflict, coercive parenting, or even physical abuse of children, as well as for children with autism, anxiety disorders, and social phobias. However, as a set of life skills, CBT has potential benefits that reach far beyond these realms. CBT has been shown to be as effective as medication for treating anxiety and depression in children, reducing behavioral problems, raising self-esteem and academic performance, and preventing substance use and improving mental health in teens.

All day long, we are fighting against faulty or unhelpful ways of thinking and learned patterns of unhelpful behavior. I think we can all agree on that. So these are all thought holes that get in our way each day. But we can disrupt them by learning to recognize our own distortions (thought holes) and then reevaluate those thought holes in light of reality. It's like when you recognize you are in a dream: all of a sudden you have the power to defeat the monsters. We can work with our kids to teach them to hack their own brains too, helping them figure out how to use their problem-solving skills to cope with difficult situations. And the more you (and they) do it, the more you develop a greater sense of confidence in your own abilities. *Boom!* You've just disrupted the brain with self-awareness through the use of CBT exercises, which we'll get into later in the book.

Mind Hack Level 2: DBT aka CBT thought hole disruptor with Buddha's superhero cape on

CBT is the broader umbrella therapy. Dialectical behavior therapy, or DBT, is a spinoff for more severe personality issues or extra-sticky thought hole patterns in the brain. It's like the difference between a regular at-home dental flossing and a dentist's office professional cleaning—but for your brain. DBT is more hard-core. How so, you ask? With DBT, Buddha is brought into the mix! If CBT and Buddhism had a baby, it would be DBT. So think of DBT as Buddha therapy. My hat goes off to Dr. Marsha Linehan, superhero psychologist and the creator of this gold standard therapy technique. She is my favorite hero, second *only* to Ruth Bader Ginsberg. Dr. Linehan combined the core tenets of CBT with Buddhist principles such as acceptance, mindfulness, and tolerating distress.

Buddha therapy is my secret weapon

I really can't stress enough how awesome this Buddha therapy (DBT) is—it's simply amazing in its effectiveness. I run groups for teens to teach them how to practice DBT. Parents are astounded at the progress teens make in these groups in dealing with a variety of issues, from cutting themselves to anxiety, self-esteem issues, depression, and social skill deficits. Because DBT is aimed at helping individuals regulate their emotions, it includes core tenets that I have found immensely valuable in my psychiatric practice while working with children, teens, and their parents. And why is regulating emotions so important? Because teenagers, for one, are so emotionally *dysregulated* (moody!), and they need these skills. For parents, mindfulness practices can help you calm yourself in times of crisis or when faced with the misbehavior of your child, while they can help your child cope with negative emotions and build healthy self-esteem. Sometimes I run the groups with parents and children together, so they both learn the skills and can practice them at home. The emotional regulation skills in Buddha therapy can help your teen find their wiser mind, calm down, and arrive at more rational decisions. As I mentioned before, Buddha therapy can also teach you and your teen interpersonal relationship skills so you can get along better with each other and the world around you.

To be right, or to be effective...

• • • •

As mentioned at the very beginning of this book, the relationships you have in your own life–how you treat your parents, your partner, and your friends–are the models for your children's future relationships.

It is very important that you create relationships that are as positive as possible in order to reflect these onto your children. Ask yourself if getting your point of view across in a fight with one of your own parents, for example, is as important as remaining calm when it comes to how you are perceived by your children. When confronting the question "Is it better to be right or to be effective?" choose to be effective–every time. Sometimes you need to give up a fight when your child is watching in order to demonstrate kindness and compassion. Being an effective parent means taking into consideration other factors, such as how the fight will ultimately affect your child. Remember that your child is always watching and someday they will repeat your mistakes, so do your best not to make them.

Passing down the wisdom

Own it!

Owning your sexual story is another great way to be a role model to your child. It's not about just your past experiences, or what went wrong, or what things you regret; it's about weaving your story into a narrative that you can rely on. Your sexual story is an amalgam of what you learned about sex from your parents, elders, and teachers, past relationships, sexual experiences, books, and everything that left an impression on you about sex.

Weave it!

It is important to weave what you have learned and what you wish you had known into a sexual narrative that you can pass on to your child. This is part of the transmission of wisdom from those who came before us–something that is desperately lacking in Western cultures! It is called intergenerational wisdom. I have seen so many examples from other cultures of tribal elders, or wise older people, passing on their experiences about life, love, and sex to their children and grandchildren. I see so little of this in our country today. Think of movies like *Moana* or *Coco*, or rituals like bat mitzvahs, or Native American coming-of-age ceremonies, or communities like Tamera in Portugal (described later).

The passing down of narratives comes so easily for other cultures but is lacking in our own. I have learned that incorporating what is best from many parenting cultures is ideal for the creation of a sexual story.

Share it!

So, parents, again I must proclaim: Don't awkwardly ad-lib with that sex talk at age 12. Don't just wing it! Plan this story out. Take the wisdom handed down from your elders (parents, grandparents, and other wise family members) and use it to create your own sexual story. Then share your story with your child to help them as they start building their own narrative.

Parenting styles & strategies
• • • •

Now that I have convinced you of the importance of addressing the topic of sex as a parent, I want to give you a foundational understanding of various overall parenting strategies and explain which one has the best outcome. As you already know, I believe that parents in any familial arrangement can be successful at child rearing—just as parents in any familial arrangement will make mistakes. Raising children is not easy for anyone. At the same time, different parenting styles and strategies can have a huge effect on a child, impacting cognitive development as well as social, psychological, and sexual adjustment.

Psychologists recognize several core parenting styles, differentiated by the amount of behavioral and psychological control parents exert over their children and the emotional nature of the parent-child relationship: authoritative, authoritarian, permissive, and neglectful.

Core styles

Authoritative parenting "is characterized by high levels of emotional warmth, support, and responsiveness, and communicating expectations in a manner that is firm, democratic, and transparent." This is the type of parent you should strive to be (and reading this book is starting you down that path!). This style gets 12 stars from me!

Authoritarian parenting, on the other hand, "is characterized by a lack of emotional warmth and support for the child, non-transparent declaration of rules, and high levels of control." In other words, meet "Tiger Mom" (as portrayed in the book *Battle Hymn of the Tiger Mother* by Amy Chua), a strict and demanding form of parenting. Tiger parents push and pressure their children towards attaining high levels of achievement.

Permissive parenting is characterized by parental indulgence that, while emotionally nurturing, ultimately creates an environment without enough structure for children to develop self-discipline. Permissive parents sometimes run the risk of placing their children in the role of parent (parentifying) but not setting appropriate limits. Often, children are asked to care for themselves in a way they are not ready to handle developmentally.

Neglectful parenting is potentially even more harmful to a child's development, as these parents show so little practical or emotional engagement that the child will experience lasting difficulties building social relationships and succeeding in school. These parents may expect the child to become an emotional caretaker, and attend to the parents' needs in the case of divorce or trauma.

Core outcomes

Parenting styles have been studied in relation to both the externalizing (acting out) and internalizing (feeling sad) effects on the child. Children of both authoritative and authoritarian parents exhibit fewer overt behavioral problems than those of permissive or neglectful parents, for example, because their parents are engaged in a "hands-on" approach to monitoring their child's behavior and enforcing rules. These children know what is expected of them and how their parents or other adults will respond. Authoritative and authoritarian parents differ in *how* they enforce rules, however. A strict requirement to obey rules with little explanation of why the rules exist—and enforcing these rules punitively—comes at a cost to the child. Authoritarian parenting has been associated with increased externalizing effects, such as aggression towards peers and noncompliance with parents. Children with authoritarian parents may also exhibit internalizing effects such as depression, anxiety, fearfulness, and low self-esteem, and have been found to be less proficient at emotional self-regulation and moral reasoning. Authoritative parenting, on the other hand, involves balancing the child's needs for both nurturance and firm limits in order to obtain optimal psychological development.

Key Takeaway:
Authoritative parenting is believed to lead to optimal psychological development.

· ·

The forbidden toy

In his classic "forbidden toy" experiment, psychologist Jonathan Freedman examined preschool children's responses to threats of punishment. In the experiment, a child was left alone in a room and told that they could play with any toy in the room *except* the battery-operated robot. One group of children was threatened beforehand with punishment (a valuable would be taken away) if they played with the robot; another group received only a mild threat (they wouldn't receive a gift). Most children in each group resisted the urge to play with the robot. The more interesting results came a few months later, when the children were brought back into the same room under different pretenses—same toys, no threats. The children who had been more severely threatened originally were now *more likely* to play with the robot, while the children who had received a mild threat avoided it. A threat of punishment is highly effective when that threat is likely to be carried out by authority figures. Milder prohibitions, however, increase compliance over time because the child devalues the forbidden object or activity. Rather than being forced to behave in a prescribed manner, the child convinces themselves that a certain behavior is preferable.

I have seen this play out in my practice over and over. Take away their phone for a week and children quickly forget about the punishment, and behavior doesn't change when they get the phone back. Take it away for a day and they are longing for it back and will be more likely to comply.

The long-term effects of Tiger Mom authoritarianism

Would you respect or listen to your boss if they were unreasonable and punitive? Or if they never followed through on their threats? No! You would probably just try not to get caught but do what you could to make your own decisions.

The effects of a parenting style last far beyond childhood. Studies have found links between parenting style and peer relationships in adolescence. Among behaviorally inhibited children, harsh, authoritarian parenting styles were later associated with diminished cortically based cognitive flexibility in the types of distressing social interactions common to adolescents. In other words, your adolescent kid is not going to be as well equipped to handle difficult interactions with their peers. Adolescents with authoritarian parents may also eventually rebel against the strict control, turning to peers for advice, support, and moral guidance. Adults who were raised by authoritarian parents report more depressive symptoms and poor psychological adjustment.

Key Takeaway:
Give a punishment that is short in duration and explain the reason for the punishment, and your child will listen.

• • • • • • • • • • • • • • • • • • • •

The dark side of the negative

One might also think of parenting styles as comprising constellations of positive and negative parenting *strategies*. Negative disciplinary strategies include behaviors such as yelling, force or physical punishment, and emotional withdrawal when faced with a child's misbehavior. In terms of communication, negative strategies include taking a "top-down" approach, such as withholding information, nagging, criticizing, or expressing hostility, disgust, or other negative affects. Negative, high-conflict parenting is associated with increased anxiety, depressive symptoms, aggression, and decreased self-esteem and school satisfaction. Negative parenting has also been associated with higher levels of sexual activity among teens.

"Do as I say, not as I do" doesn't work

Social learning theory, developed by Albert Bandura, proposes that we learn by modeling the behaviors, attitudes, and emotional reactions of other people. In several classic studies conducted at Stanford University, he found that children readily imitated the behavior of adults, even when those adults were no longer present.

One study, for example, involved nursery school children who watched adults model play behavior with toys, including a five-foot inflated "Bobo," or clown doll. One group of children were exposed to an adult who played with Tinkertoys, ignoring the doll. Another group of children were exposed to an adult who acted aggressively towards the Bobo doll, kicking, punching, and sitting on it. When the children were then allowed to play with the toys alone, those who had watched the aggressive adult tended to imitate his or her behavior towards the doll, even with significant time lapses between sessions.

Children watch and imitate their parents even more closely than they imitate other adults. Correlations have been found between parents' displays of negative emotions and children's ability to regulate their own emotions, and between marital aggression and children's difficult relationships with peers. Corporal punishment, a negative disciplinary strategy associated primarily with an authoritarian parenting style, increases the probability that a child will exhibit behavioral problems and antisocial behavior. Children who are hit for misbehavior learn that dealing with conflict involves aggression. Aggression can thus be transmitted across generations. Women with childhood experiences of physical abuse or aggression are more likely than other mothers to spank their infants, for example.

Focus on the positive

Positive parenting strategies, on the other hand, focus on reinforcement of good behavior rather than verbal or physical punishment for bad behavior, clear and consistent communication, and healthy emotional relationships between parents and children. When children are behaving acceptably, parents offer verbal or nonverbal praise. If a child is noncompliant, the parent should offer and repeat clear instructions, praise attempts at following these instructions, ignore the child rather than yell, and if necessary (and appropriate for the child's age) use a "time-out." A time-out allows your child a moment to reflect on their own about their behavior and takes away any reinforcement you or others may have unwittingly been giving them for their bad behavior.

Positive communication means providing clear instructions rather than insinuations or questions that could be confusing to the child, and responding consistently each time an issue arises. Positive communicators also use verbal and nonverbal expressions of respect, warmth, and affection such as hugging or praising, along with responsiveness–attentiveness to the child's physical and emotional state and at least some level of support or recognition of the child's desires. This interchange between the parent and the child can become more active "give-and-take" or negotiation as the child ages.

Among families with children exhibiting behavioral problems, positive parenting strategies have proven effective in curbing children's deviant behavior. Positive parenting techniques have also been found to improve parental attitudes towards difficult children, reduce parental stress, and even reduce the possibility of future abuse in abusive parent-child dyads. An abusive parent-child dyad refers to a situation where there is a poor fit between parent and child. This would be the case, for example, with a depressed mother and a hyperactive child, where the mother lacks the skills to deal with the child's hyperactivity and resorts to screaming or hitting instead.

Key Takeaway:
When parenting, think positive.

Studies have shown that adopting an authoritative parenting style and positive parenting strategies makes it possible to set and enforce strict boundaries for a child's behavior while remaining respectful, loving, and attentive to the child's needs. There are even parent training programs you can attend to help you develop positive parenting strategies and authoritative practices. Parent training programs, which focus on positive reinforcement, staying calm, ignoring outbursts, and enforcing time-outs, are an extremely effective way to reduce behavioral problems. Studies show that parent training programs have resulted in better outcomes for children, reducing externalizing behaviors (outbursts, etc.) and internalizing behaviors (self-hatred, avoidance, etc.), improving cognitive outcomes and social skills, and keeping children in school and out of the criminal justice system.

I have used parent training with the families of my patients with oppositional or externalizing behaviors and have found it to be very effective in reducing these behaviors. Children don't come with instruction manuals . . . but I have one to offer you, and it works.

Positive parenting styles repeatedly win over negative parenting styles when it comes to enhancing a child's educational achievement, self-esteem, independence, emotional regulation, perspective taking, and social competence. The American Academy of Pediatrics has hardened its stance against spanking and corporal punishment as a mounting body of evidence correlates corporal punishment with negative psychological outcomes.

You can easily incorporate sex positivity into your overall positive parenting strategy

The foundation of great parenting is an authoritative parenting style, giving clear guidelines and discipline but allowing your children to make their own decisions whenever possible. So, now that we've made the case for positive parenting overall, we can tie that underlying strategy into how we approach your child's burgeoning sexuality: just stick to the positive. Your child's decision to have sex is not something you will ultimately be able to control, so I hope that as a parent you can foster a positive relationship so your child can come to you with concerns.

Parents, I want to give you the tools to provide reasonable boundaries, explanations, and guidance for how your children should behave. Being authoritative doesn't mean threatening them with harsh consequences if they act in a way you don't agree with. Try to help them come to the best decisions for themselves on their own, rather than force them to behave as you want them to. The latter course of action will just make them more subversive. Give them the tools they need, then unleash them on the world to embrace their sexuality, and they will make good choices and learn from their mistakes.

2

Teaching about Bodies through the Stages

· · · ·

PARENTS SOMETIMES WORRY that a child is "not ready" for information about sex, and admittedly, children do develop at different rates. Yet if you pay attention to your child's burgeoning cognitive abilities and tailor your discussions in the ways suggested in this chapter, your child will learn about sex in the same manner that they learn about cooking, geography, or football.

Information about sex is thus presented gradually, naturally, and in a way that is integrated with everyday life. Rather than being a topic that requires a special time and place to be discussed, sex is dealt with when it comes up, immediately and without inducing shame. Providing small pieces of information in casual conversations will prove far more beneficial over the long run than anxiously preparing for a single "Talk."

Instead of having the mother talk with a girl and the father talk with a boy, as many did in the past, all parents should play active roles in sex education, whether they have conversations with a child separately or together. And although it may seem as if boys and girls should be educated on slightly different topics, it is beneficial to provide them with as much information as possible about how both male *and* female bodies work, regardless of which body they inhabit. "Period boy" was a middle schooler who caused a media sensation when he posted a video on YouTube suggesting that women would not need tampons if they learned to "control their bladders." He was widely mocked, but the episode made it clear that boys in many age groups do not understand what menstruation is or how it happens. Girls should gain an understanding of how the male body works as well.

It's "vulva" not "peepee": teaching about bodies from birth to 7 years old

• • • •

Birth to two years old is the first stage of cognitive development. Piaget termed this the "sensorimotor stage," as children begin to develop muscular skills and to differentiate themselves in the world. By age two or three, most children start developing a sense of gender identity and social awareness along with their language skills. Some children adopt stereotypical gender interests—donning princess dresses or carrying fake guns and light sabers—while others remain more neutral. Either way, decisions about how to dress or what games to play are important experiments for toddlers.

Avoid reinforcing the social constructs of gender

Parents should avoid reinforcing harmful gender stereotypes, allowing children to explore a range of toys and clothing. Children will imitate the behaviors and gender presentation of adults in their lives. By age four, children are on their way to more advanced forms of reasoning, and engaging in symbolic thinking and imaginative play. Although birth to four years is a time of immense cognitive development overall, one's approach to sex education can generally remain focused on a few basic concepts.

It's your vulva! Vagina! Anus! Penis! Testicles! And other terms to use unabashedly

Children should be taught the proper terms for their genitals from the time they can *understand* language. Even before your child is talking, use the proper terms for the genitals rather than slang or "cute" terms that are vague and idiosyncratic. Instruct other caregivers to do the same. Be aware of the language used at your child's preschool or day care, and alert the staff to your preferences. Both girls and boys should learn terms such as "vulva," "vagina," "anus," "penis," and "testicles." If you haven't been using them, start right away. Naming body parts can prevent sexual abuse—and a study of 91 sex offenders of children shows that they would avoid children who knew the correct names of their body parts. Toilet training should also involve correct terminology and accurate explanations of bodily processes. This is also a good time to teach children how to clean themselves—wiping front to back, washing hands, and so on.

What can happen when you don't educate at this stage?

A Patient's Story: Laura

ONE OF THE YOUNG girls in my practice, a seven-year-old named Laura, licked her friend Kathy's vulva during a playdate. Kathy was upset and told her parents, who in turn told Laura's parents. When questioned, Laura explained that she had heard that adults did it to each other to have fun, so she wanted to try it. Laura's parents angrily asked her, "Where did you learn this?" Laura shut down, refusing to tell them that she had heard about it from her older brother. The next day at school, Laura also refused to speak to Kathy because she had gotten her in trouble, making the situation worse.

Laura was referred to me for evaluation. I found that Laura was not troubled, but simply uneducated in matters of sexuality, bodily autonomy, and boundary setting. Her parents had not talked to her or her brother about bodily autonomy, or told them that they should not touch anyone else's genitals. I suggested that Laura's parents talk about sex with her, explaining that she could think about doing these things someday, but that for now she was not allowed to touch anyone's private parts except her own. They needed to teach her the correct terms for body parts and point to exactly where they were on the body: "penis," "vagina," "vulva," "anus," "nipples." I asked Laura to apologize to Kathy the next day, both for touching her and for not speaking to her. To smooth things over and repair the friendship, I proposed a trip for ice cream. Luckily, Kathy's parents were understanding, but things could have gone quite differently if they had not been.

What should you do if your child touches someone else inappropriately?

- Don't panic. Many times, this is a part of normal developmental play. Lack of education around boundaries is likely the reason. Speak to your child to determine why they did it or where they learned about it. I have seen this happen because an older child touched them first or was playing a sexualized game. It is important to find out all about the incident before reacting. Most of the time it will be enough to give the child the education they need to prevent it from happening again.

- Speak to your child about the incident and the importance of never touching anyone else's genitals. Make sure they understand exactly what you are saying; name and point to the body parts on their body where they shouldn't touch others.

- Consider if the child is being adequately supervised, if they are over at someone else's house or under another caregiver's watch, to ensure their/others' safety.

- Tell the parent/parents of the other child(ren) involved and make sure they address it with their child(ren) and get the help they may need.

- If you feel this behavior is very concerning or part of a pattern of behavior, make sure you talk to a professional/authorities. This may be an indication of a previous history of sexual abuse or trauma. (See below.)

What should you do if your young child says that another child or an adult touched them inappropriately?

First, ask questions. You may need to ask how they were touched and ask them to show you. If the story seems credible–given that young children are limited in how well they can explain such things–you should approach the other person to get another perspective on the story. If the contact was with another child, you could ask them, "Did you touch his penis?" or ask them where the touches occurred and why. Most commonly, one finds a sibling or cousins spanking each other or showing each other their genitals. You will want to repeat your explanations of bodily autonomy without undue shaming.

If you are concerned about sexual abuse occurring with an adult, you will want to carefully weigh your options. Do not panic, especially in front of your child. It may make sense for your child to see a child psychiatrist or therapist to assess what occurred and whether they have experienced trauma. You will also want to remove your child from any possible interactions with the individual who may have acted inappropriately.

Even as you remain alert to possible violations, realize that not every inappropriate touch is the work of a pedophile or a cause for severe alarm. Sometimes, it is instead a signal that more education and discussion is necessary. There are many good resources that delve into this subject more deeply if you have specific concerns about your child.

Tips that can minimize your child's risk of molestation

These tips come from the American Academy of Pediatrics.

- In early childhood, parents can teach their children the names of the genitals, just as they teach their child names of other body parts. This teaches that the genitals, while private, are not so private that you can't talk about them.

- Parents can teach young children about the privacy of body parts, and that no one has the right to touch their body if they don't want that to happen. Children should also learn to respect the right to privacy of other people.

- Teach children early and often that there are no secrets between children and their parents, and that they should feel comfortable talking with their parents about anything—good or bad, fun or sad, easy or difficult.

- Beware of adults who offer children special gifts or toys, or adults who want to take your child on a "special outing" or to special events.

- Enroll your child in day care and other programs that have a parent "open door" policy. Monitor and participate in activities whenever possible.

- As children get older, create an environment at home in which sexual topics can be discussed comfortably. Use news items and publicized reports of child sexual abuse to start discussions of safety, and reiterate that children should always tell a parent about anyone who is taking advantage of them sexually.

- If your child discloses any history of sexual abuse, listen carefully, and take his or her disclosure seriously. Too often, children are not believed, particularly if they implicate a family member as the perpetrator. Contact your pediatrician, the local child protection service agency, or the police. If you don't intervene, the abuse might continue, and the child may come to believe that home is not safe and that you are not available to help.

· Support your child and let them know that they are not responsible for the abuse.

· Bring your child to a physician for a medical examination to ensure that the child's physical health has not been affected by the abuse.

· Most children and their families will also need professional counseling to help them through this ordeal, and your pediatrician can refer you to community resources for psychological help.

Stick to the facts

During these early years, even very young children may ask questions about male and female bodies and try to figure out where babies come from. (See "8 things to know about nudity" on page 54 for thoughts on how to handle nudity in your home.) Pregnancy often sparks questions, and provides a good opportunity to have conversations about the differences between men's and women's bodies, and between children's and adults' bodies. There are many good books to guide a discussion on pregnancy, such as *What Makes a Baby* by Cory Silverberg, *It's Not the Stork!* or *It's So Amazing!* by Robie Harris, and *Your Story: IVF* by Kylie and Mathew Hill. Some children find pictures of a developing fetus to be interesting and helpful.

Explanations should be factual, but not necessarily more detailed than the child requests. Explaining that a baby grows in the uterus, which is like a sack of muscles that holds the baby safe while it grows, is both accurate and calming, for example. Do not explain reproduction using stories about "the stork" or a baby coming out of "Mommy's tummy," as these explanations can cause fear. Further, even if your child is initially accepting, the next phases of cognitive development require them to reject fanciful explanations. A parent's answers should be aimed at preventing rather than furthering confusion. If a child asks a question that surprises you or seems "out of the blue," you may want to ask what they have already heard from peers or teachers or what prompted the question.

Figure out the "why"

Understanding *why* the child is asking can help you decide how to initially answer the question and how much detail is appropriate. A child might ask if two women can have a baby, for example. The scientific answer to such a question could be a bit overwhelming to a preschooler, but if you learn that another child at school has "two mommies," you can frame your answer to address your child's concerns. They might indeed be wondering about the mechanics of reproduction; however, they might also simply be wondering about the logistics of Father's Day or about who does household tasks.

Providing information on how "the sperm and the egg" meet to start the process of making a baby is appropriate if your child is curious, although not every child will want to know exactly *how* the sperm and egg meet. If your explanation is accepted without further questions, you have given enough information for the moment, without resorting to euphemisms. Some children may return several months later with more questions: "But Mommy, you explained about the sperm and the egg, but *how* does the sperm get to the egg?" Aha! It's the million-dollar question you have been waiting for—and possibly dreading. Realize that if your child is asking the question, they are ready to know the answer.

One of my clients had a seven-year-old son who had heard from a teacher at school during a sexual education class that babies were made through sex, and that sex involved a father's sperm meeting a mother's egg. He asked his mother, "Is this what you and Daddy did?"

When she replied, "Yes, that's how we had you," he shook his head and said, "You must have been glad when it was all over!" In fact, she replied, they *were* glad, as sex feels good. A few weeks later he wanted the rest of the story: "Mommy, how does the sperm meet the egg?" She explained that when the penis rubs together with a vagina, sperm is released; the sperm has tails that allow it to swim inside her up into the uterus to fertilize the egg. Good job, Mom, for being factual!

Whatever the age at which the question is posed, you should answer with more facts: "The sperm comes out of the penis of the man, and the egg comes from the ovaries of the woman." If the child still wants to know more, a deeper explanation is possible, while pointing to the appropriate points on the body: "The man rubs his penis inside the woman's vagina, the sperm comes out, swims up to the uterus, and finds the egg. When the sperm meets the egg, they combine and start to grow into a baby. This is called sex, and is something that adults do when they are ready." Most children will save these questions for when they are older, but it is always smart to be prepared.

Keep it #casual

When parents develop relationships with their children that involve ongoing communication about sexuality, it is natural to provide more details as a topic arises again or your child requests more information. Develop a habit of talking informally and with ease about bodies and reproduction before shame or shyness make such topics difficult to broach at later ages. If you experience discomfort using words like "vulva," "vagina," "nipple," or "penis," this is a good time to begin saying those words out loud and in casual conversations with your child. Children are not born uncomfortable with these discussions, so it is good to take advantage of their openness.

Address masturbation

Some children begin masturbating during this time, which is normal. For very young children, under four years, the best approach is simply to ignore the behavior. Exploring their bodies is normal and healthy, and any comments about it can create shame. Older children can be told that "touching your penis or vagina is normal and can feel good, but it must be done in private." You can also explain that it is not appropriate for them to show or ask anyone else to touch their genitals: "It is okay to touch your vagina and vulva [or penis] when you are by yourself. However, you must touch only when you are alone and not allow anyone else to touch unless it is me or Daddy/other caregivers. If anyone else touches you there [point to the exact areas], tell me/other caregivers right away."

According to the book *Beyond Birds & Bees*, Bonnie Rough writes that in Amsterdam, for children, it is all about the dos. Children can masturbate and experience pleasure whenever they want; it's up to the parents and other adults to take on the don'ts. "Don't look at a child who is masturbating." "Don't tell the child not to touch themselves in public, it will create shaming." This approach assumes they will eventually figure out that doing so in public is not commonplace. This radical acceptance of public behavior is more extreme than I would practice. I believe it's a good idea to say to your child, in a very calm, very frank tone, that it's best done when they are alone. Don't let them see your discomfort.

Children are taught to wash their hands after using the toilet, and may or may not assume that they should do so after touching their genitals for other reasons as well. Given that these areas are sensitive, children might be instructed to wash their hands *before* touching their genitals as well. Pinworms—tiny parasitic worms that live in the gastrointestinal tract—are still commonly spread in preschool and elementary schools. Eggs can be spread from person to person through contaminated fingers or clothing, as when children do not wipe properly or scratch their anal area and then interact with other children. As when wiping after urination or defecation, children should be instructed that touch should always proceed from front to back. The message should be to wipe from front to back to prevent germs and to always wash your hands after going to the toilet.

Fact fix! Teaching bodies to 7- to 11-year-olds

• • • •

During the early elementary years, children move through Piaget's "preoperational stage," increasing their capacity for symbolic thinking and logical reasoning. Children are very imaginative during these years, relying on intuition more than abstract conceptual thought processes. Between ages 7 and 11, the stage that Piaget referred to as the "concrete operational stage," the child's thought processes mature. The egocentric perspective of early childhood is tempered with a developing understanding of the emotional states of other people.

Meet your child where they are

Children do not progress through developmental stages linearly or on the exact same timeline. However, noticing how your child responds to and processes new information can help you interact with them. Children in the preoperational stage, for example–who are egocentric and still unable to use logical and abstract thought to solve problems–will deal differently with a divorce than children who have moved into the concrete operational stage. Children in the preoperational stage may be most concerned with how a divorce will affect their everyday life, such as where they will live or what bed they will sleep in afterwards. They will not show significant concern for their parents' emotions.

Seriously, just focus on the facts

Sometimes, different types of reasoning can be layered onto the same situation. A friend's daughter was in first grade when the family dog died. Her mother at first said that the dog had been "put to sleep." This is a euphemism–an innocuous word to replace words that may sound more painful or offensive. Confused, the daughter asked, "Well, when will she wake up?" Her mother then had to explain that the dog had in fact died. The daughter's first response to this news was anger at her mother: "Why would you tell me that? That is a horrible thing to say to me." Her mother was surprised by the reaction, but responded by saying, "I'm sorry to tell you, but I thought that if your friends asked where he was, you would want to know." The girl's next response was to exclaim, "Can we get a new puppy tonight?" When her mother said no, that first she needed time to feel better about losing this pet, the girl began to express sadness over the loss.

It would have been easier if the mother had just told her the dog had died to begin with. If a child cannot grasp euphemism, saying that a pet was "put to sleep" may be even scarier than it is comforting. Even for children growing up in religious families, psychologists suggest coupling religious explanations with biological facts. For example, you might explain that the pet's body stopped working properly and it died *before* God took it to Heaven. Children who are not provided with this type of information may believe that they could fall asleep and never wake up, or that they might be "put to sleep" by parents, God, or another force.

These same guidelines apply to euphemistic explanations of sex or reproduction. These can be similarly confusing, such as referring to "making love" rather than having sex, or labeling body parts with cutesy terms. All of this can create more confusion for your child, and should be avoided.

Dispel the playground theories

Children sometimes create their own theories about sex and reproduction and share them with each other. If your child questions your answer, or presents an incorrect explanation, you can ask how they got their information. Teachers, caregivers, or other children may use slang words for body parts (calling a penis a "willy," for example) or offer "cute" or misguided descriptions of sex. A friend's child heard from one of her peers that babies were made when the father urinated inside the mother; correcting such a factual error is important even if further information is not being requested at the time.

Explain reproductive options

This might also be a good time to introduce the idea that biological reproduction is just one of several ways that babies can be made. Some children will want to know more, while others will already be on to the next topic. (For more information about how to explain artificial insemination, adoption, in vitro fertilization, or other related topics, see chapter 7.)

Explain menstruation

Young boys and girls at this stage may notice tampons or maxi pads around the house or on television. Parents can explain what these items are for as soon as a child discovers them, using a simple explanation like, "These are used by women after puberty." If the child sees blood on a tampon, maxi pad, or underwear, more detail can be given: "After puberty, when the body is ready, teenage girls and women make a little bit more blood. This blood would help a woman's body to make a baby, but if it is not needed that month, the body gets rid of it. It doesn't hurt." If the child is a young girl, assure her that it will not happen to her for many years.

Explain birth

Some children grow up around animals, seeing them go into "heat," have sex, or even give birth. These children may have a greater understanding of how sex works than their peers, if their parents have been forthcoming with the correct information, but they may also have more detailed questions. Children may also be exposed to sex in the animal world during trips to a zoo or farm. Answering questions factually is important to avoid instilling fear in the child. It may be appropriate to explain that human mothers will have options to prevent them from feeling too much pain, and that they usually have doctors in attendance to make sure the baby comes out healthy.

Explain sexual threat and boundaries

Children at this stage should be informed about the dangers of sexual assault and violence. They will be exposed to media stories and potentially hear more personal accounts. Media attention to certain high-profile cases can be used to spark discussions. Although we cannot protect ourselves completely, being clear about our own personal boundaries and having the confidence and skill to enforce those boundaries can help us avoid many uncomfortable situations.

Empower your child by helping them think through how they might respond in dangerous situations. Taking a self-defense class as a family can also help build confidence.

Rapid changes: teaching bodies approaching puberty
• • • •

By middle school, ages 7 to 13, your child has entered the concrete operational stage. Their thought is less egocentric, more socially oriented, and increasingly logical and abstract. They can study more advanced symbolic or abstract concepts, such as algebra and science, and consider multiple outcomes for hypothetical situations.

Your child may also be approaching puberty. By puberty, your child will be undergoing rapid physical changes as well as changes in cognitive development. Hormones surge—not just the sex hormones that lead to the development of secondary sex characteristics, but also hormones related to pair bonding, such as oxytocin and dopamine. The visible development of secondary sex characteristics is accompanied by important psychological changes, such as early struggles for independence and experimentation with new identities. During this phase of adolescence, boys and girls are figuring out what kind of adults they want to become.

Be sensitive and respectful
Children mature at different rates, with some preteens still looking and behaving like middle schoolers while others are developing secondary sex characteristics and undergoing personality changes. Recognize and respect the major changes your child is experiencing.

Explain the changes to come
Middle schoolers of both sexes should know about the types of bodily changes they can expect as they enter adolescence, both for themselves and for opposite-sex peers: the growth of pubic hair and arm hair, the development of breasts, the beginning of menstruation, and so on. If they have seen naked adult bodies and asked questions all

along, they will already know and be prepared for the changes to come (see page 53).

Developing a healthy body image begins earlier than middle school, although this is a time when issues may become heightened due to the physical changes of adolescence, peer relationships, and media influence. Some children suddenly become uncomfortable with sports or other activities they used to enjoy due to the development of secondary sex characteristics.

Focus on health, not appearance

Parents should take care to model a healthy relationship with their own body, as well as try to steer the emphasis on their child's appearance towards health rather than attaining cultural ideals. The middle school years are an ideal time for both parents to model healthy habits, such as exercising and eating well, and to have discussions with their children about beauty ideals. (See also the self-image exercise beginning on page 243.)

Give them the HPV vaccine NOW

Targeted interventions in sexual and reproductive health are increasingly recommended for early adolescents, ages 10 to 14, as well as later adolescents and young adults. The Centers for Disease Control and Prevention (CDC) and many pediatricians now recommend that 11- and 12-year-olds receive the HPV (human papillomavirus) vaccine. Parents should familiarize themselves with the latest research and information on the control of HPV, which can lead to cervical or throat cancers. Although HPV is considered a sexually transmitted infection, recent studies have suggested important nonsexual means of transmission as well. Because most people are eventually exposed to HPV, vaccinating before someone engages in much skin-to-skin contact with others is believed to be beneficial.

You are going to need to get more proactive at this stage

As your child may be more reticent to initiate discussions at this stage, parents should be proactive. Every so often, preteen sexuality becomes a media topic. Some media stories are sensationalized. "Rainbow parties"–parties where groups of young girls wearing different colors of lipstick supposedly gave oral sex to boys–turned out to be an urban legend after being reported on *Oprah* in 2003. The "choking game" of more recent years, however, which was practiced by some preteens and adolescents as a novelty or an autoerotic practice, resulted in some actual deaths around the country. Media attention to sexuality presents an opportunity to bring up these topics with your child. Ask whether they have heard about the practice or incident being reported. Ask if their friends have talked about such things, and how they reacted.

Stay one step ahead: teaching bodies at puberty and beyond
• • • •

By high school, your child is on the way to becoming an adult. Piaget's "formal operational stage," which ranges from 11 or older and lasts until about 15 to 20, depending on the individual, marks the maturation of cognitive thought processes. An individual becomes capable of hypothetical and deductive reasoning, testing hypotheses, and nuanced causal explanations.

Teenagers vary in their responses to the changes of adolescence. Even if your child has always shared with you, you may find that as a teenager they suddenly become reticent to talk. The responsibility for starting a conversation about sex–or continuing the conversation that you began in infancy–is likely to fall on your shoulders as a parent.

Stay involved in ongoing communication about sex
Most parents would prefer that their teenagers delay sexual initiation, whether for religious, health, psychological, or other reasons. What is the perfect age to start having sex? Because most teens have not finished with puberty and are still developing, the maturity level of most children is such that they are not equipped to handle the emotions

that will ensue. Another issue is that, legally, the age of consent for sexual activity is 16, so that sex between one person who is over 18 and another who is under 16 may be viewed as statutory rape. For girls, an earlier introduction to sexual activity may predict depression. For both males and females, it may be associated with alcohol use, multiple sexual partners, and STIs. I realize that teenagers mature differently, both physically and emotionally. More important than set-ting a specific age for sex is keeping the communication lines open. Try to be involved in this discussion, as this will lead not only to more thoughtful experimentation by your teen but to safer practices. (More about this in chapter 5.)

Stay up-to-date on their sexual activity

Parents should question their teen about which sexual activities they are engaging in. Asking questions is of course the most direct way to begin assessing how sexually active your teenager is: "Have you ever been kissed? Who was it?" or "Was it a boy or a girl?" You can move on from kissing to sexualized touching. It may be easier to talk about "private parts" than to use more formal terms like "penis" or "vagina" (or, better yet, find out how teenagers are referring to sexual activities such as "going down on" or blow jobs). If direct questioning is unsuccessful, there are other ways to initiate an exchange. Indi-rect questions—such as "What do you and your friends think about 15-year-old girls having sex?"—can open up a more personal conver-sation. Find out what the hot new Netflix series is among teens, and familiarize yourself with the issues it raises. Specific scenes or char-acters can be brought up to start talking about uncomfortable issues.

Stay up-to-date on their social media platforms

Show an interest in their social media profiles—and don't assume they use the same sites that you do! Find out how social media is being used by teens. A post or a photo can spark a discussion about how teens are expected to dress or behave. (See chapter 6 for additional informa-tion on how to keep kids safe on social media platforms.) Remember not to impose your own thoughts or values on the post, but rather let your child speak about their thoughts and ask open-ended questions such as, "Do you think it's possible that post might be Photoshopped?" or "Do you think that dress a bit revealing for a day at school?"

Prepare them ahead of sexual activity

Even if you would prefer that your child wait to become sexually active, it is best to prepare them with accurate information based on the assumption that they will gain sexual experience during high school. For girls who are sexually active or thinking of becoming sexually active, this is a good time to set up an appointment for a first gynecological exam or appointment with the adolescent medicine doctor rather than a pediatrician. Although you will want to give your child some privacy with the doctor during the appointment, setting the stage for the discussion and finding the right doctor is the parent's job. Don't be daunted: You read reviews and talked to other parents to find them the best dentist, the right pediatrician. You can do this.

Cover condom importance and best practices

Condom use and contraception are essential topics to cover with both sexes—even if your teen tries to reassure you that intercourse is not on their agenda. Condom use is important to teach and stress even for a teen who is taking oral contraceptives or using other forms of birth control, as it can minimize the risks of both STIs and pregnancy. Condoms, when used correctly, are 97 percent effective at preventing pregnancy. Your teen needs to understand how to use a condom properly, and to make sure to remove it immediately after ejaculation to prevent leakage. Improper use leads to accidents. Parents should educate their teens on best practices with condoms.

Cover birth control options

Be open to discussion about birth control. Birth control is not giving your child permission to have sex, but helping them to make smart and healthy decisions about their body and future. Backup forms of birth control, such as birth control pills or an IUD, can be used alongside condoms. There are many types of birth control pills on the market today, designed to minimize side effects and work with an individual's needs. Some oral contraceptives can help control adolescent acne. Many of my teen patients have benefited from an IUD, which is easy to insert after they become sexually active. An IUD is effective without requiring any additional responsibility on the part of the teen. The traditional copper IUD has potential negative side effects, such as bleeding or scarring upon removal, and is only offered to teens who have already had children. In recent years, new types of IUDs, such as the three-year lower-hormone Skyla (approved for teens) and the five-year Mirena, have been developed that release a tiny amount of progesterone into the tissues around the uterus. The progesterone fools the body into thinking it is already pregnant and stops ovulation—like traditional hormonal birth control but with fewer side effects. These devices are easily inserted into the cervix during a basic pelvic exam, and later removed via a small string. In addition to being relatively painless, the IUDs cannot be felt during sex and reduce periods to very light spotting. The hormones can help with acne and mood swings as well.

My amazing local pediatrician (Dr. Gail Schonfeld in New York) has even started inserting them. She told me recently during a visit with my children, "It's not enough to walk around with my signs and to support women's health. I need to start practicing what I preach!" She must be one of the few pediatricians who perform IUD procedures for teens. I appreciate her talking to kids like my daughter about sex after politely asking me to leave the room so they can have a frank doctor-patient discussion. We need more frontline pediatricians like her—preventing pregnancy and helping teens be sex-positive.

Another thing to note: if your teen is LGBTQ+, you'll want to address both condoms and birth control in ways that are particular to them, as the risks may still be there and preventing them still matters.

Educate them about STIs

Teens should gain an understanding of the various sexually transmitted infections and how to protect themselves before they become sexually active. Many school sex education programs cover STIs in the curriculum, although you may also need to discuss the symptoms of bladder or yeast infections, something that school programs may leave out.

Do not forget to talk about pleasure!

In addition to the dangers associated with sexual activity, remember to address sexual pleasure as an important component of sexual health. Dr. Debby Herbenick, an amazing sex researcher for Kinsey Institute, explains that 30 percent of all women and 7 percent of men experience pain during sex. This is a stunning fact. Do you want your child to be one of these stats? Of course not! Explain to your teen that sexual pleasure starts with understanding their own body. Masturbation can teach them what types of touch feel comfortable, the pressure needed, and the timing of each phase of arousal.

Suggest that a good relationship will involve conversation between the partners about what feels good, and if such conversation is avoided or shut down, the relationship should probably not become even more intimate. If a person is mature enough to have sex, they should be mature enough to have conversations about what they do and do not like, and what their boundaries are. Encourage them to be honest about what feels good and what does not. Concern for a partner's sexual pleasure can be expressed even by those who are sexually inexperienced themselves.

Discuss ways to start such conversations with a partner. Making a joke could be productive in some situations, for example: "Okay, I'm not sure what I'm doing down here, can you help me?" Also let your child know that if sex is painful, you are there to help and will make sure they get the guidance they need to figure out what is the matter.

In my practice, I ask all the teens I work with who admit to being sexually active or sexually curious about their experiences of intimacy and pleasure. If they won't answer, I prod by saying something like, "If you can do the crime, you can do the time [with me]." I ask about their own experiences with orgasm, but I also ask boys if they have ever given a girl an orgasm and, if so, how they did it. It's always surprising to me how many girls say they do not have orgasms, or even pleasure, during sex. Some even say that they are only having sex because they fear that if they do not, their boyfriend will dump them. I also ask about masturbation, and whether they would feel comfortable showing their partner what works to give them pleasure. Usually, they squirm or refuse to answer! But once the seed has been planted, I know it will grow. They realize that deeper communication with a partner can enhance everything about their experience.

Give your kid more credit

I realize I am in a unique position in relation to the teens in my practice, and that parents cannot expect to be privy to the same disclosures. However, most parents do not realize the depth of the conversations they could be having with their teens. Parents can be a great resource, offering information and guidance on many of these topics, if they are able to overcome their own reservations about discussing sex.

There is more on this topic in chapter 5.

The full monty: teaching bodies throughout the stages
• • • •

One topic that deserves special attention throughout all the developmental stages is nudity in the home. Getting naked with your children promotes a body-positive self-esteem.

Furthermore, it can help your child embrace their body throughout the life cycle. I see a lot of fear in children (and of course in adults) about growing old. People are going to great lengths to look younger and are never taught about the aging process and invited to embrace it. We see people undergoing crazy, painful, and expensive plastic surgery. This may be a little off topic for this book, but I do believe some of our culture's obsession with youth and fear of getting older is due to the fact that we never see older people naked, and rarely see older people featured in a positive light in the media. We are taught to idealize youth and to fear getting older. This has led to many people disfiguring their bodies in an attempt to look young, as well as developing severe depression and self-esteem issues as they get older.

Is this what you want for your child (or yourself)? Best we embrace it head-on, and teach our children that growing older is nothing to be afraid of. Wrinkles mean that each line has developed through time and experience, and older people have so much to offer this world and should be cherished for the wisdom and memories they have accumulated. Death is the last great transition; if we avoid it, it will still come for us, and it can be a beautiful experience. We should put more effort into dignifying it, and not distance children from the dying. Instead, allow death to be a lesson for them. Part of the problem is that children are sheltered from caring for the elderly, and never see them naked. This is a mistake. (See the Power 9 section in chapter 4 about how the happiest cultures embrace their elders.) Why not organize a full family skinny-dip including Grandma/Grandpa? This way, they can see the full spectrum of the aging process, and learn that sagging, wrinkly skin is just the next iteration of age. European families have a much more open attitude towards nudity than Americans—and also have less fear about getting older.

8 things to know about nudity

1   **Be explicit about the fact that there are different cultural rules around nudity.** How nudity is handled varies across cultures and even across families. In some northern European communities, whole families will hot-tub together naked. In Germany, some public pools allow kids to swim naked until the age of six; adults may frequently strip down on beaches or in parks. Elsewhere, however, we find numerous restrictions on when one can undress and in front of whom. Explaining such differences to children will help them develop an understanding of appropriate behavior in their own cultural context, as well as an ability to refrain from judgment when faced with different customs or beliefs.

2   **Be explicit about situational rules as they come into play.** Being naked is normal in some situations and inappropriate in others, even within your own family. When children are young, they have not developed a sense of modesty based on cultural prescriptions, and do not care who sees them naked. Eventually, though, a child will need to manage the display of their body in

expected ways, and parents can help children learn to do this without instilling a sense of shame. During the early years, you can create opportunities for them to see you naked. You may want to bathe together, as they will need help anyway. Request privacy when you want it, however, as when using the toilet. Children should also learn that nakedness will make people uncomfortable in some situations, such as when visitors are present. Nakedness will be natural and expected in some places, such as in the bathroom or bedroom when changing, but out of place, for example, in the kitchen.

3 **Set patterns and expectations early.** Opposite-sex nudity within the family is not unacceptable or traumatizing if it occurs early and in appropriate contexts, for example. For straight or gay men raising daughters in the US, for example, male nudity will not be shocking if it was treated as normal during the early years. The same goes for opposite-sex siblings (although care should be taken from very early on to teach siblings to uphold stricter boundaries when their friends are present in the home).

4 **It's okay to politely compare bodies and ask questions.** Develop a sense of ease and comfort with your own body and with responding to questions. Your young children will look at your body, comparing it with their own or with your partner's body. They may ask questions about breasts, penises, or pubic hair, and parents should respond factually (breasts provide milk for babies, hair provides cooling protection because adults' bodies are warmer, etc.). This process also teaches children when it is acceptable to look at other people's bodies and what types of comments are appropriate.

5. **Use nudity as a teaching moment.** Teach your child the correct name for each body part: penis, vagina, vulva, breasts, buttocks, etc. Learning the proper words will aid in their understanding of anatomy and cut down on confusion. It will also keep your child safer. If a child learns to differentiate between body parts, he or she will also be able to differentiate between appropriate touches.

An accidental touch on the buttocks during play is very different from someone attempting to touch the vulva–but if this whole area is referred to as a "bum bum," the child will have difficulty both interpreting and communicating about the behavior of others. With older children, nudity can also spark conversations about the changes to expect during adolescence.

6 **Keep eroticism out of the picture.** Being naked, even with a partner present, does not mean that it is okay to be sexually expressive. Do not rub or touch a partner in sexually explicit ways, as this may confuse a young child.

7 **Follow the child's lead.** By adolescence, self-consciousness about nudity usually develops regardless of how a child was raised. Some adolescents may want to accompany a parent into a steam room naked, or go skinny-dipping with the family, while others will not, even if they were okay with it in the past. Respect such decisions, and use cues to determine their comfort level even if nothing is stated directly. Some children may be uncomfortable with either their own nudity or yours in earlier years as well. Honoring a younger child's feelings can be done in sex-positive ways, for example by going along with requests to bathe separately at a certain age but not to hide your nakedness in your own bedroom or the bathroom.

8 **Cultivate lifelong attitudes.** Comfort with one's naked body translates into healthy behaviors later in life. Confidence, self-esteem, and body image are intertwined. Your child is watching how you respond to changes in your appearance or health, how you handle aging, and the ways in which you are influenced by cultural ideals of beauty, masculinity, or femininity. Notice if you criticize your own appearance in front of your child. Even if you lack self-esteem, you do not necessarily need to pass that on. When appropriate, talk about the differences between the bodies you see in magazines or on television and the body that you have. Frame behaviors such as dieting in terms of health rather than just appearance.

3

Teaching Boundaries, Consent, & Privacy

• • • •

SEX-POSITIVE PARENTING is not just about sex; it's also about relationships. You are teaching your child ways of interacting with others. The social importance of developing an understanding of boundaries and consent runs far deeper than sexuality. It is not just a "no means no" approach, but speaks to the boundaries we set on our personal lives, extending to our deeper views on love and relationships.

This chapter explains how to approach this continuous conversation and education with your child about boundaries, consent, and privacy though each developmental stage.

Teaching about boundaries

• • • •

Keeping your child safe from unwanted physical advances is a process that starts early in life, from the moment they learn the proper terms for their genitals and about appropriate interactions with others. Ideally, boys and girls should learn how to avoid unwanted contact with others long before high school, but the conversation about boundaries and consent should be revisited regularly. Another reason to address boundary and consent issues both early and often is that consent is a pressing legal concern. Schools, camps, colleges, workplaces, and other environments are taking sexual harassment and consent violations very seriously. Parents should, too.

Some of the events unfolding recently in the news–for instance the debate about sexual harassment claims of consent violations made by celebrities, medical professionals, and CEOs—raise the issue of personal responsibility. Why didn't the young girls violated by Dr. Larry Nassar report his behavior? Why didn't people in positions of authority believe them when reports were made? Some of the explanation lies in power dynamics, and the use of fear and manipulation that enforces silence. But some of the explanation also lies in how we are raising our children.

Teens may be aware of the fact that they can say no if they do not want to participate in a given activity, sexual or otherwise, but true empowerment means having the ability to overcome guilt, fear of being disliked, or worry about displaying bad manners. True empowerment means being able to say, "Get off me, you're a creep," without fear of social repercussions. From their early years, young girls need to learn how to interact with men from a place of strength. This is one of the reasons I truly believe that young women should have a variety of male role models in their lives. Admittedly, many men are reluctant to take on such roles, due to the contemporary legal climate; they limit any conversation to their own children or avoid the topic altogether. But such conversations can be truly life-changing. This topic is explored in more detail in chapter 4.

Body bubbles: teaching boundaries from birth to 7 years old
• • • •

Even very young children can begin to learn boundaries by observing how their parents deal with their behavior, such as touching others' body parts, grabbing hair, or opening doors without knocking. They can also learn to express their own feelings about being touched, whether positive or negative.

The bubble trick
The idea of a "bubble" around the child's body may help them express their feelings if they do not want to be touched or if another

child is acting aggressively towards them. Parents can model the use of a bubble if a child is pulling their hair or jewelry, kicking, or otherwise entering their space inappropriately, indicating with their hands, "This is my bubble, do not enter it." As children develop an understanding that other people have similar mental states, they learn respect for others' boundaries as well. The "bubble" can extend to accepting items such as food or toys from strangers. Children can be taught to ask a parent or caregiver before accepting such items into their personal bubble.

If you have a family pet, interactions between the pet and your child can further serve as an example of personal boundaries. Even children without pets, however, should be taught that dogs, cats, and other animals require respect. Children should not pull tails, ears, or fur and should notice an animal's discomfort before being confronted with a snarl or growl or hiss. Most dogs and cats show obvious signs when they feel threatened–ears pulled back, teeth showing, cowering, shaking or shivering, and so on–before they become aggressive. Point out the animal's body bubble, and help your child pay attention to both warning signs and requests for contact, such as rolling over on its back, rubbing against your legs or body, or following you. Such training not only prevents bites, scratches, and more dangerous injuries, but it also teaches the concepts of bodily autonomy and boundary management.

Give them permission to say no

Parents can explain that parents, doctors, and caregivers may at times need to touch them, but other people, whether children or adults, should not be touching the child's genitals. Give the child permission to say no if they are uncomfortable with something. This could be as simple as "my body no touch," or invoke the idea of time–"no touching now." (Obviously, there are limitations, as when a diaper needs to be changed!)

If your child wants to kiss or hug another child–even at ages younger than two–they should first ask: "Can I kiss you?" or "Do you want a hug?" You can model this behavior by asking your child if you may kiss or hug them and waiting for their response, or asking permission to wash various parts of their body or to adjust their clothing (even if you are going to need to step in anyway).

Respecting boundaries and teaching consent also means that children should never be forced to engage with anyone physically if they do not wish to, except in situations such as a medical emergency. Requesting that your child hug, kiss, or otherwise touch another child or adult–even close family members–teaches them to ignore their own feelings in favor of "politeness." Less physical alternatives can be offered, such as a fist-bump, a high-five, or even a wave.

When your child can communicate with words, ask that they share experiences with you that made them uncomfortable or that were inappropriate. These discussions should not be used to instill unnecessary fear but to reinforce the idea of bodily autonomy. Some experiences that make a child uncomfortable may indeed be appropriate– a doctor's appointment, for example–but learning to talk about these feelings creates a foundation for later discussions. Similarly, introducing the idea of consent at a young age translates into greater comfort with the idea later.

If you have a child with disabilities or a nonverbal child, remember that they often still hear you, and absorb the message, even if they can't tell you as easily when something feels wrong. Stay consistent in your messaging and don't be afraid to repeat it.

Teach your kid to be radically inclusive and resistant to peer pressure

The term "radical inclusion" is the first principle of Burning Man, which means to be welcoming to others, including strangers, as well as being open-minded and nonjudgmental. If everyone taught their children to be inclusive of their peers, including people they don't want to be friends with, there would be little bullying. However, this does not mean you have to invite everyone to take part in everything you do; it just basically means being kind to everyone, even when people are not kind back. And of course this does not mean you have to give in to peer pressure. During the elementary years, children become immersed in a world of peers in addition to ongoing relationships with caregivers. Addressing peer pressure at an early age is important, and a discussion can be framed in terms of boundaries. Even elementary schoolers may pressure each other to touch, harass, or exclude a peer, and should be reminded that doing so may have ramifications beyond what their friends claim. Explicitly encourage your child to stand up for their friends in bullying situations and to befriend less popular peers. Books like *Wonder* by R.J. Palacio are aimed at this age group and can spark discussion about compassion. Children can learn a great deal from inclusive birthday parties (where every child is invited, regardless of popularity) or being asked to socialize across groups.

Standing up to peer pressure in elementary school becomes a foundation for autonomy in later years. If kids learn to say no when they do not want to do something minor that another child requests (going down the slide backwards, sneaking candy, or making fun of a friend), they will be more likely to say no in adolescence to bigger requests that do not feel right. This is a skill that may delay sexual initiation and prevent them from ending up in situations where they are at risk for sexual assault.

Playing "house"

During the elementary years, children usually pair off and play mostly with their own gender. As this is an imaginative phase, children may act out scenes of a sexual nature, make their dolls kiss or go on dates, or mimic behaviors they observe in adults. Children may play "boyfriend" and "girlfriend" with each other, for example, or play-act with family roles (mother, father, baby). Making sure that your child understands and respects bodily boundaries will prevent such play from progressing too far.

Make personal autonomy a habit

If you have developed a habit of addressing issues naturally as they arise, it will not be difficult to reinforce the basic ideas of personal and bodily boundaries, moving from simple metaphors such as the bubble to actual statements of autonomy: "Please don't grab me. It's my body and I get to decide who touches me." Allow your child to express pleasure or dislike with certain types of touch, and respect their wishes. Some children do not like to be hugged or tickled, while others crave it. Allowing your child to express an opinion about whether they want to be touched in their early relationships gives them permission to continue thoughtfully saying yes or no throughout their lives.

Parents should caution against any nonconsensual contact with other children. "Wedgies" (when underwear is forcefully pulled up), "pantsing" (when pants are pulled down to expose underwear or genitals), or playful spanking will no longer be seen as harmless when they occur on school grounds. Parents should also model restraint themselves, however. Tickling, "blowing raspberries," or other types of play can be done in ways that teach children passivity *or* bodily autonomy. Children should never be held down and forced to submit to a parent's–or sibling's–game.

Be aware of gender bias in your interactions

Parents should also be aware of how their own gender biases may affect their interactions with their young children. Fathers are more likely to roughhouse with sons than daughters, or to "play-punch" as a sign of bonding. Yet *any* such touching without explicit consent, even that which is meant to be playful, can indicate that boys have implicit permission to touch others as they wish. Parents should also model behavior that does not rely on manipulation or ridicule.

We must constantly be aware of how we use forms of "pressure" to persuade others to act in certain ways. For instance, your child will notice if you engage in gossip or act "fake" towards other adults, just as they will notice if boys and girls are treated differently, and they will inherit your bias.

The rebellion begins! Teaching boundaries to 7- to 13-year-olds

• • • •

As your child grows, they will spend more time without parental supervision. You will want to make a point of raising these issues around bodily autonomy as specific occasions approach (mixed-sex parties or sleepovers, school dances, summer sleepaway camp, etc.).

Sensitivity, privacy, and rebellion!

You may notice that middle schoolers become sensitive to even minor boundary violations. Preteens may shy away from hugs or kisses from parents or relatives. They may feel awkward changing clothes in front of friends or siblings. Some middle school children begin to desire complete privacy for bathing and changing. This development is healthy and signals a burgeoning independence. Of course, this is also the time when rebelling against a parent becomes a natural progression in the development of a unique sense of self. Middle schoolers who act responsibly can earn more freedom on playdates or when alone in their room. However, parents must still monitor their behavior to ensure that rules are obeyed.

Experimentation with intimacy

Even young middle schoolers may begin experimenting with intimate contact with peers, from holding hands to kissing or progressing through the "bases." Games like Spin the Bottle or Two Minutes in the Closet may be a part of the social scene regardless of what you are advocating at home. Sex-positive parents will differ on which types of contact are tolerable at which ages. Some parents may believe that these experiments are normal, and will want to explain that holding hands, kissing, or nongenital touching is acceptable if it feels good and the child does not feel pressured. Other parents may be more comfortable forbidding these behaviors altogether. Realize, however, that making a behavior punishable necessarily impacts your child's willingness to discuss it in the future.

Reinforce the right to refuse touch

Continue to address nonsexual body violations–bra strap snapping, purposeful tripping, pinning the arms, pulling hair, etc.–to reinforce the idea of autonomy and consent. Reinforce the idea that everyone has a right to refuse touch, and that this message can be delivered firmly. If asking a peer to stop does not work, an adult can be asked to intervene.

Your child should also be given the right to refuse touch from other adults, even parents and family members. Allowing them to express their feelings is healthy, and develops communication skills that can be applied in many future situations. Assure your child that you will not punish them for asking questions or seeking help if they feel pressured or uncomfortable in any situation. Also, remind your child that some types of contact could be problematic if they do not seek consent first.

With a deepening understanding of and respect for bodily autonomy, obtaining sexual consent will eventually become a natural extension of proper manners. Many parents teach their children that displaying good manners reflects on the reputation of the family. Interacting politely with others, doing good deeds, avoiding gossip, showing gratitude, being respectful when accepting or declining invitations, and showing kindness and respect to people–even if you do not like them–are considered social obligations and ways to make your parents proud. Why, then, do parents not have similar conversations with their older children about how to treat intimate partners?

Addressing sexual desire

At this stage, parents can start talking about how to handle sexual desire. Desires to masturbate or think about sex are normal, and children can be assured that they are healthy. This is also an important time to discuss the reasons for waiting to have sex. Explain that physical and emotional maturity are necessary for sex to be a healthy experience. Explain that having sex too young could be unsatisfying or even physically or emotionally uncomfortable. Explain that waiting until you are in a relationship with someone who cares about you, on the other hand, can make the first experience special and safer. Reassure your child that you will be there to answer questions at each step along the way, rather than simply stepping back and letting them wonder if the time is right.

Get real & get legal: teaching boundaries during puberty & beyond

• • • •

Remind your teen that they can say no if they feel pressured into sex, substance use, or other activities.

Explain the legalities

Pay attention to situations that could leave you or your teenager legally culpable. Explicit consent has become a legal standard in many contexts, and should be practiced by teenagers. Asking directly–"Can I kiss you?" or "May I touch you there?"–may be the safest approach for your teenager to take in their intimate interactions with peers. Young men should be exceptionally careful to obtain explicit consent for any intimate encounters and to make sure that their partner is not intoxicated, although young women should also think about these issues.

Depending on where you live, legal issues can arise if there is an age difference between teenagers who are dating, even if their sexual activity is consensual. It is important to repeat these conversations even if you had them in middle school; remind your teen that it is never appropriate to take nude photos or share them through email, text, or mobile applications. Child pornography laws may apply to sexting between teenagers–even their own selfies! Be clear that this is a *legal* issue. Even downloading or forwarding a photo sent by someone else can leave one legally culpable. States have also created statutes for the prosecution of "revenge porn," which can sometimes be very broadly interpreted (see chapter 6). Do not assume your teenager knows how to handle these situations, or even understands the complexities involved.

A Patient's Story: **Libby**

A PATIENT OF MINE named Libby recounted a story of how her mother's advice helped her navigate a tricky situation in eighth grade. She went to a high school party with friends, and was thrilled when a popular sophomore boy started paying attention to her. She shared a beer with him. Eventually, she found herself kissing him in a dark bedroom. He tried to take off her shirt, but she said no. A few minutes later, he placed her hand on his jeans so that she could feel his erection, saying, "You have to help me with this or I'm going to feel really sick later." She removed her hand. They kissed again and he placed her hand back on his pants. "You don't want to give me blue balls, do you?"

The phrase triggered a memory of a conversation she'd had with her mother before school started. Her mother had warned her that someone might try to pressure her to go further than she wanted. "If a guy tells you that he's going to get 'blue balls,'" her mother said, "all you need to do is remind him that he can take care of the situation just as easily as you can. He's already been using his own hand for years." "Oh, Mom, do we need to talk about this?!" Libby had replied with embarrassment at the time.

But now, in a social situation where she might have had difficulty expressing her feelings, her mom's words offered her a quick comeback. Not only did she not accept the guilt, but she responded, "No, I don't want you to feel sick. But I know that you can take care of it just as easily with your own hand as mine." Laughter erupted from the closet, where several other sophomore guys were hiding. Libby was mortified, but then realized that not only had her mother's advice given her permission to say no when she did not want to go further, it had also saved her from a difficult situation.

Parents deserve privacy: teaching privacy from birth to 7 years old
• • • •

Introduce parental privacy

Cultivating a balance between openness about sexuality in the family and individual privacy is important. Obviously, infants and toddlers cannot be granted a large sphere of privacy. However, by around age two, most children can understand a parent's need for privacy. Parents can ask for privacy when using the toilet by asking the child to play with their toys outside the bathroom door, for example.

Just as a parent should prepare to lock up dangerous items or place them out of reach of a small child, it is never too early to also begin preparing your home for your young child's curiosity about other parts of your life (not to mention that there is value in keeping your personal erotic toys, books, or photos away from the prying eyes of future babysitters or nannies). Locking drawers or cabinets now will create a habit of being conscious of monitoring your child's access to your personal items.

Co-sleeping

In general, I am not a fan of co-sleeping for children if it can be avoided. It can cause many issues. It does not help foster intimacy (SEX) for parents, and a healthy parental sex life is a great benefit to children in the long run. It also can become an issue when the parents are ready for the child to sleep alone, or if the couple divorces and one parent begins dating again, as the child can be resentful of the new partner who they feel kicked them out of Mom or Dad's bed.

Teaching privacy to 7- to 13-year-olds
• • • •

Privacy as a concept can similarly be expanded upon during these years. Middle school-age children can read, and should be taught to respect signs and warnings: Do Not Enter, Privacy Please, etc. If your child decides in turn to hang a sign on their own door–such as No Parents, or No Girls Allowed–you can do your best to nurture these early desires for privacy in a safe and responsible way. You might say, "Okay, that's fine unless you hear my secret knock."

Establish parental privacy

Request that your child ask permission before going into your room, digging through your purse, or exploring the contents of your mobile phone. Some children will ask questions about locked drawers or closets. You can explain that parents have things they want to keep for themselves, in the same way a child might want to keep a secret diary.

Do NOT allow privacy when it comes to the Internet

One realm where I do not recommend allowing privacy is with your child's access to the Internet. The Internet can be a great resource for children, but you should monitor the sites they visit. Despite the best parental–and technological–supervision, some things can fall through the cracks. My friend had installed software such as Qustodio and Net Nanny (parental monitor software programs) but was shocked when she heard some unsavory comments being made by the cartoon character SpongeBob. Although her daughter was too young to realize she'd unwittingly stumbled onto a SpongeBob clip that had been pornographically altered, my friend learned the limits of trusting algorithms to filter content for her child.

Answer questions right away

If such a slip occurs, instead of panicking, explain that certain videos are inappropriate for children. At young ages, the child will probably quickly be interested in the next clip anyway. If your child does see something that upsets them, or is old enough to realize the inappropriate nature of the material, be sure to handle questions the moment you discover what they have seen. As always, leave the door open for future questions as well. Answer truthfully. If they were watching sex, then say that sex is "what adults do when they get older to connect and because it feels good. You don't have to worry about that for a while." Assure your child that they can ask you questions without getting in trouble–and stick to your word. The explanations you give, even if you don't feel completely confident, are still probably better than the ones they will get from other kids or online.

Explain what not to share outside the family

Privacy extends to early discussion about what can be shared outside the family. Not every stranger is a friend or can be trusted with certain information–phone numbers, addresses, details about who lives in the house, etc. Barring emergency situations, such as when a child is separated from their parents and must approach a stranger for help, children should learn to ask their parents or other caregivers before divulging such information. In emergencies, suggest that your child first approach a police officer or other authority figure, if possible; if not, approach an adult woman with children.

Explain the WHY behind family privacy

Part of educating your child includes discussing what is and is not appropriate to share with people outside the family. Children should learn the difference between lying and maintaining boundaries and privacy. In my practice, I have described this as the difference between being right and being effective. A child who tells people the truth about themselves or their family is certainly right in doing so. But sometimes the truth is less effective than an answer that does not make people feel uncomfortable or leave members of the family open to bullying, ostracization, or other consequences. If you have been having ongoing conversations about privacy with your child, broaching this topic will be natural, even if the topic itself can be quite complicated.

The repercussions of sharing different types of information vary. In the US, gay marriage is now legal, but there are situations where same-sex/polyamorous/transgender or other out-of-the-box parents face real legal challenges in terms of issues with custody of their children. Social change is uneven. I saw on the news that a gay couple had received hate mail in their wedding RSVPs from the printing company. Children with nontraditional parents are sometimes bullied or teased, or may be left out when it comes to playdates or birthday parties, and this may depend on the community where they live. There may be situations where nontraditional parents want to share their situation and others where they may not. Having a discussion about this with children in a developmentally appropriate way can be useful. The decision about whether or not to disclose may depend on the situation in which they find themselves, as well as the parents' and their children's feelings (see the section on blender, banner, and chameleon families in chapter 8).

What can you do if your child walks in on you having sex?

• • • •

This is every parent's nightmare. Although it is normal for children to go through developmental stages where they engage in sexual exploration or flirtatious behavior, it is important for all adults and older siblings in the house to maintain appropriate boundaries. Children should never participate in, or watch other family members engage in, sexual behavior. Lock the bedroom door. Turn on loud music so that nothing you're doing can be heard outside the door. Lock your sex toys in a safe. But still, what if your child accidentally walks in on you having sex?

If you make it a big deal, they'll make it a big deal

How you handle the situation, of course, will depend on the specific circumstances, the age of the child, and the relationship you have built up to that point. Do not scream or get angry, or act ashamed; what you're engaged in is a normal thing, and it's nothing to be ashamed of. Kids pick up immediately on your emotional reactions, and the weirder you act, the more fearful or "grossed out" they will be.

If you've established boundaries that allow for privacy, the first response would be to address why those boundaries were overstepped. Was there a knock on the door? Was the door supposed to be locked? Reiterate the importance of respecting adult privacy, but also acknowledge your own responsibility if you forgot to lock the door or didn't realize that school was letting out early.

If a young child walks in, say, "Please go back to your bedroom. We are fine, but we need privacy right now." The incident may be forgotten, but if they ask later what you were doing, answer honestly: "We were having sex, which is what grown-ups do when they care about each other. But we need privacy, so that is why we lock the door or close it. And that is why you should always knock." Hopefully, your child will already understand what sex is, but if not, this is definitely the time to broach that topic!

Inform the other parent

The situation becomes far more complicated if your child walks in while you are with someone they would not expect. Young children should never be asked to keep secrets for a parent, even in situations with potentially dire consequences, because they are psychologically unprepared for such a responsibility. Even if you are going through a divorce, you should always be the one to inform the other parent if a situation like this arises. You will also need to explain to your child that you are sorry they found out about a complicated adult situation in such a way, that you made a mistake, and that you meant to introduce the relationship in a different way.

After the initial shock has passed, you may want to plan an outing to introduce the new partner in a completely different environment–going out for ice cream, visiting a park, or going to a local fair, for example.

4

Happy Humans! Helping Kids Form Healthy Relationships for Life

· · · ·

TEACHING CHILDREN about sex is one small piece of a much greater public puzzle. What we really want is for our children to be happy. Happiness comes from forming stable relationships. Harvard's landmark study of adult development, studying 75-year longitudinal data, shows that happiness is directly correlated to forming intimate relationships. So what's the overarching lesson from this study? Good relationships keep us happier and healthier. Period.

So guess what? It's not only about your wealth, your genes, your success... The biggest predictor of your overall happiness and fulfillment in life is, basically, the presence of love.

This is not just the finding of this one study, but an important and well-researched finding of any study ever done on happiness. Take the Berkeley happiness project, a Greater Good Science Center initiative that focuses on happiness. (They have a great online course on happiness, by the way, and healthy relationships are a focus.)

When we look at the "blue zones"—geographic regions where people live the longest—such as Okinawa, Japan, and Sardinia, Italy, certain things are constants, including healthy social relationships. One healthy social habit found in blue zones in particular was that even if people were feeling grumpy, they still walked outside their homes each day and spoke to many different people who knew them personally. As a result, if there was a change in their mood or health, it would be immediately noticed by others. So basically, people in those blue zones were constantly in each other's business—and this was a good predictor of psychological well-being and health! This requires that you develop and maintain good relationships.

The Power 9
• • • •

Author Dan Buettner has an amazing list called "The Power 9" in his book *The Blue Zones: 9 Lessons for Living Longer from the People Who've Lived the Longest.* He says, "To make it to age 100, you have to have won the genetic lottery. But most of us have the capacity to make it well into our early 90's and largely without chronic disease." The "blue zones" are areas where people regularly live to 90 and beyond. Buettner teamed with *National Geographic* in a study, and they uncovered nine evidence-based common denominators among the world's centenarians that are believed to slow the aging process.

There's much to learn from the nine categories, and to me they can also be applied to raising healthy kids and modeling better behavior ourselves. For example, the idea that *exercise happens naturally*: the world's longest-lived people are not forcing exercise; they move around their environment naturally, and exercise is part of their lifestyle and community—such as tending their gardens or walking to neighbors' houses. Similarly, we could choose to take the stairs or walk to work, and thereby make exercise a normal part of every day, rather than force ourselves to spend time at the gym, which we often forgo when stressed or busy.

Buettner stresses *purpose*, which translates to "why I wake up in the morning." Knowing your sense of purpose is worth up to seven years of extra life expectancy. For me, knowing I wanted to help children has given me a real sense of direction in my life.

Buettner also talks about the need to "downshift," which I interpret to mean stress management. He says, "Stress leads to chronic inflammation, associated with every major age-related disease. What the world's longest-lived people have that others do not are routines to shed that stress." Consider adding yoga, meditation, or an afternoon siesta to your day. Many schools are now incorporating yoga as a regular activity or break between lessons, and it is also used by occupational therapists with special needs students since it can put kids more in touch with their bodies and emotions.

Good eating is important too. Eat the most in the morning. Buettner reminds us of the Okinawan 2,500-year-old Confucian mantra *"Hara hachi bu."* It is "said before meals [and] reminds them to stop eating when their stomachs are 80% full. The 20% gap between not being hungry and feeling full could be the difference between losing weight or gaining it." What I tell most of my patients is that when you eat natural foods, it is much harder to overeat because the fiber in natural foods stimulates your satiety reflex. So if you're eating naturally, chances are you will stay thin and healthy, and so will your children. However, packaged foods full of salt, sugar, and other additives to stimulate appetite override your body's natural instincts and lead to obesity. People in the blue zones eat naturally and stay healthy without much thought to weight.

Buettner talks about "Plant Slant. Beans, including fava, black, soy, and lentils, are the cornerstone of most blue zones diets. Meat—mostly pork—is eaten on average only five times per month, and in a serving of three to four ounces, about the size of a deck of cards." That tried-and-true Mediterranean diet promotes the best brain health and cancer prevention. There is also a recent study that shows teenaged girls who eat more fiber are less likely to get breast cancer when they're older—so push fiber on your girls!

Be a wino (within reason)! Moderate drinkers outlive nondrinkers. One to two glasses per day with friends is okay—for you, of course, not your teen! But I do think drinking a glass of wine at dinner on special occasions with your teenagers can be a great way to expose them to healthy drinking patterns rather than letting alcohol consumption be a forbidden and therefore taboo activity that might turn into bingeing later on.

Buettner brings up so many ideas that I think are important to how we (and our kids) live. One of his categories is "Belong," which means being part of something greater than yourself. Being part of faith-based or community-based organizations can improve life expectancy. He writes, "Research shows that attending faith-based or community services 4 times per month will add 4 to 14 years of life expectancy." I interpret this to mean that any kind of community-centered involvement can be important to your family; if it's not religion, it can be participating in your neighborhood organizations or school-based community organizations. Or see later in this chapter, where I talk about creating rituals for your family that can help promote a sense of belonging for your kids. These rituals can be one-off or happen every year as part of the development of self-esteem.

Buettner writes about putting loved ones first. Taking care of one's family includes the elderly. He also talks about the "Right Tribe." I interpret this as the family you choose. "The social networks of long-lived people favorably shape their health behaviors," Buettner writes.

Adapting your family life to embrace community is crucial. It's not just the family you are born with that's important, it's also the family you choose. Creating community within your family's social life will engender a positive kind of peer pressure that will help keep your kids in check and prevent bad or risky behavior. In my experience, nothing is more effective for nurturing good practices than a teenager who has great, caring friends who give them good advice. This always counts more than any advice I, or their parents, provide.

So, parents, work hard to create a beautiful, balanced community around your family. This includes exposing your children to families with good values and creating opportunities for positive mentoring relationships with the people in your world who you think can be great influences on your child. I have gone to great lengths to ensure my children have spent time with amazing businesspeople, athletes, families from different racial and ethnic backgrounds, the LGBTQ+ community, and so on. The goal is to create a community that will inspire them but also look out for them. With my own children, I find that challenging the right people in their lives to mentor them has been incredibly powerful, and creating opportunities for my friends to get involved and help educate my children has resulted in enormous positive change for them. I encourage all parents to do the same.

So, what do Buettner's blue zones teach us? That what we want for our kids is for them to form bonding relationships with long-term partners (which provides stability), and to prioritize family and social relationships so they can live long, productive lives with minimal exposure to the stress hormones that can kill them. Not to mention healthy eating and exercise. All of this is accomplished by promoting a healthy relationship between our children, their bodies, and the world around them. We need to give them the tools to love themselves, and to have great interpersonal relationships with both their family (you, the parent) and their future lovers and friends. So, parents, create "blue zones" around your home and family. Love and sex are intimately connected when it comes to our romantic relationships, but healthy relationships in general are the main topic of this chapter.

The need for a primary caregiver

Babies must attach to a primary caregiver, no matter what sex or gender. This is a very important developmental stage. Daily attention from a primary caregiver is essential, and outsourcing this parenting time to a nanny can be psychologically detrimental to the child. If a 10-month-old baby cries when it is taken away from its primary caregiver and put into the arms of a stranger, that is normal and healthy. If the child seems ambivalent, that is a warning sign of trouble to come.

In my ideal world, one parent, regardless of gender, would be able to take the role of "The Artist Formerly Known as The Mom"–taking three months off from work after the birth of the child to allow for this attachment process, and then cutting back on hours or taking an easier work track to spend time at home for the first year of the child's life. Same-sex and dual-career parents should consider the benefits of allowing for secure attachment in this phase of their child's life. They may want to consider who can more easily take the time off and who is better suited to the role. As a working mother myself, I am not suggesting that becoming a full-time, stay-at-home mom is the only way to raise a healthy child. But I did cut my work hours back to two days a week for the first six months, and then three to four days per week after that until my kids entered preschool. It is unrealistic to believe that one can work 80 hours a week and be the primary caregiver for a child. Hurray for modern families in which the "dad" picks up the slack if the "mom" is the higher income earner!

When you "stay together for the child"

. . . .

I see many parents in my practice "staying together for the child" with very negative consequences. There must be a balance between the parents' unhappiness in a strained and loveless relationship and the benefit that might come from "staying together." One of the most important things you can be as a parent is a positive role model. Children learn most of what they know about relationships from watching their parents navigate the world around them. The children I see with the most serious emotional issues often have parents who are poor role models: children of divorce, where the parents could not get along; children who have lived in invalidating environments and watched the parents disrespect each other or be disrespected; children who have picked up that their parents are sacrificing their own sexual needs for the sake of the partnership and are clearly living in loveless and sad states. Put it this way: if you know that you are living in a loveless and sad state for the "benefit" of a "partnership for the kid's sake," your kid also knows, and it is not doing them any good.

Many of the children I see who have grown up like this have unhealthy sexual lives or fall victim to sexual assault or painful and unfulfilling sexual experiences. Many have parents who either are uninvolved in the discussion of sexuality with their children or have been abused themselves. Most parents don't love their bodies and never get naked in the home, and don't give their child the tools to love the skin they are in.

It is very rare that an unhappy couple provides a happy, stable environment, and since being a good role model is the number one way to parent successfully, I believe that a peaceful and kind separation with major effort put into peaceful co-parenting is usually a better option.

How to incorporate the opposite-sex role model

. . . .

Becoming a positive role model requires coming to terms with your own sexual story and reframing it into an empowering and "path-forward" narrative. I provide suggestions on how to do this in chapter 8.

Lesbian couples or single moms might look among their friends or relatives for male role models who can be trusted. Gay male couples may have an easier time finding opposite-sex role models, given how many women work with children as teachers or babysitters or in other roles. However, an ongoing relationship with an opposite-sex adult is important for these families as well.

Even as your child develops, conversations about sex are best shared by all parental figures, although different topics might be assigned to each. Fathers might feel uncomfortable talking with their daughter about menstruation but more comfortable with other topics. Fathers should be reminded that this is an opportunity to show their daughter how men can be caring and respectful towards women both in their actions and with open-minded conversations. Conversation topics could be the gossip that goes on in her school, what he sees in her social media accounts, and even media figures in the news. Outrageous media events can be used as talking points. For instance, a father might condemn Donald Trump's "grab her by the pussy" comment as degrading to women. Or there was the story about T.I., a celebrity who told social media he takes his daughter to the gynecologist to check her hymen yearly to make sure she stays a virgin. A father might say to his daughter that he does not agree with the rapper, and that he would want her to come to him when she is thinking of having sex rather than hiding and being fearful he would get upset.

A mother may prefer that the father be the one who talks to their son about masturbation or condom use. However, there is no reason to shut out the possibility of a "mom"-driven conversation on other pertinent topics, such as how women's bodies work, what girls expect in relationships, or how to decide when to have sex.

There is a tendency to leave sex education to the parent who is the same sex as the child, or to divvy up the topics by the sex of the parent (mothers talk about menstruation with daughters; fathers talk about abstinence with daughters and condom use with sons). Sometimes it is useful for a child to talk with someone whose body works the same way. It could be tough for someone without a vagina to explain how a yeast infection feels or how to insert a tampon, for example. Or for someone who has never had a penis to describe the best way to remove a condom after intercourse to prevent pregnancy or sexually transmitted infections (removing it before the erection subsides, then washing oneself with soap and water). Both male and female adolescents are more likely to have discussions about sexual topics with their mothers than with their fathers, although studies show male adolescents are more comfortable talking to their fathers than female adolescents are. With that being said, there are good reasons for both parents to play active roles in this process.

The case for a "father" role model in a girl's healthy development
. . . .

In my practice, I have repeatedly witnessed the impact of a lack of opposite-sex role models, especially for girls. When I work with a young woman struggling with self-esteem or body image issues, I am not surprised to hear that she did not feel the influence of an adult male role model in her life. Sometimes I find these young women are behaving promiscuously not because they want sex or pleasure, but because they are feeling desperate for male attention of any sort.

Fathers often tend to withdraw as girls start to develop secondary sex characteristics, but they could instead take the opportunity to talk with girls about respecting their body as they grow into women.

A father should directly address unwanted touch or sexual advances when talking with his daughter, explaining that no one should touch her without her permission. Simply because he is an adult male—and, in some parental relationships, somewhat idealized—his words can have a powerful impact. Adult men become role models for how men behave in sexually intimate relationships—whether they realize it or not.

As Canadian prime minister Justin Trudeau wrote, our sons, not just our daughters, "have the power and the responsibility to change our culture of sexism." As a parent of boys, he says,

[I want] to help them grow into empathetic young people and adults, strong allies who walk through the world with openness, love, and a fierce attachment to justice. I want my sons to escape the pressure to be a particular kind of masculine that is so damaging to men and to the people around them. I want them to be comfortable being themselves and being feminists—who stand up for what's right, and who can look themselves in the eye with pride.

Fathers, or other male role models, can also have an influence on body image by explaining that men have a wider view of physical attractiveness than is presented by the media, and that a girl does not need to be stick skinny. The girls in magazines may be beautiful, but that is just one idea of beauty. Most men find curvy girls sexy, no matter what the magazines seem to put on their covers. And being attractive is not just about how much you weigh but also how you walk and dress and feel about yourself; most people find confidence attractive.

Adult men can also both model and stress that women should be treated with kindness and respect. A father can praise the child's mother for her capabilities, character, sense of humor, or other traits beyond her appearance, focusing on strength and health rather than beauty. Older adult men must obviously maintain strict boundaries. Conversations should never be personalized or include details about the parents' sex life. Saying to a daughter "you are sexy," for example, would not be appropriate, even if it could be helpful to discuss how men appreciate many kinds of women's bodies.

Don't leave out the pleasure talk!!!
• • • •

When I conducted an informal survey in my community about a man's role in sex education, most men who responded said they felt comfortable discussing reproduction, contraception, and consent. But none of them had spoken to their children or mentees about sexual pleasure, the timing of the first sexual encounter, or body image.

Both parents should cover these topics with their teens. Fathers especially should be reminded not to leave out the pleasure talk. Historically, if fathers get involved in the discussion of sex, it is usually to fearmonger ("Don't get pregnant, use birth control. If he hurts you, I will kill him"). Consent and boundaries are important components of the discussion—but it is also powerful for a father to say that a partner should prioritize sexual pleasure, and that the daughter should be enjoying sex or there might be something wrong. It's not just a case of "do no harm"; rather, the partnership should be mutually beneficial. A father can really impact his daughter's sense of self, her feeling of empowerment, and the adoption of an attitude of "taking sex," not "giving it away."

Don't leave out the consent talk!
• • • •

Similarly, mothers of sons should not leave discussions about dating or consent solely to the father to handle. A mother can shape a son's future attitudes towards women and teach him how to act respectfully and responsibly. A boy may vividly remember a conversation about consent with his mother because of their differing perspectives. A mother has a unique opportunity to shape her son's sexuality by allowing discussion beyond the typical commands ("Wear a condom, don't get her pregnant"). Why not also include a conversation about consent and pleasure? What would happen if boys heard it from their mothers first that sex would be *better*—more pleasurable, and maybe even more frequent—if they communicated with a partner? "Can I kiss you? Can I touch your breasts? Does this feel good? Am I going too fast?"

Not just the opposite-sex role model is important
• • • •

We do not need to see these differing perspectives as rooted in some sort of essential biology, but in experiences that we each have while living life in bodies that are seen as male or female by others, and treated as such. If you learn that your child does not identify as heterosexual or identifies as trans/cisgender, you will want to make sure you seek role models who have had the types of experiences your child might encounter.

Another way to think about this process is in terms of providing a variety of adult role models for your child. Many cultures relied far more heavily on extended families or neighborhoods in the business of raising children than we do today. Even if not of the opposite sex, an adult who is not a parent or primary caregiver can have a similar positive impact. We tend to discount the things that our mothers tell us; after all, mothers are *supposed* to love us unconditionally and tell us that we are beautiful, worthy, and intelligent. Hearing similar sentiments from another trusted adult can be powerful. Sometimes, approaching someone other than a parent when there is a question or problem feels easier for a child. Some families may include additional partners or stepparents who can take active roles in initiating discussions or serve as sounding boards for teens on topics that they do not want to bring up with their parents.

A Patient's Story: **Isabella**

ISABELLA, A YOUNG GIRL in my practice, was raised by a mother who suffered from depression. Isabella also had a lack of male role models in her life. Her father was much older than her mother, who was his third wife. He was uninvolved as a parent, partly because he had other grown children. He was also somewhat resentful of having to take on the responsibility of raising another young child.

Isabella came to me because she hated her body. She thought she was fat, and couldn't even stand to look at herself naked. By age 13, she started to have sex to try to get the male attention she craved. She lost her virginity in a threesome with a boy and another girl on the same night that she met them, then continued to have sex with others even though she did not enjoy it. When I initially questioned her about her sexual experiences, she was reticent. Eventually, as I persisted in my questioning, Isabella shared more details that allowed me to connect her dislike of her body and her craving for male attention. Not only did she detest looking in the mirror, but she also did not look down during sex. She also worried that if she said no to boys' requests, they would dislike her and she would be lonely. She had never had a male role model in her life tell her that she was pretty, or that she deserved to be treated with kindness and love. She sought attention through sex, rather than through friendships or accomplishments.

Later in her teen years, Isabella engaged in more violent sexual activities, allowing her sex partners—who were sometimes inappropriately older men—to spank, choke, and pinch her. When she didn't have a sex partner, she cut herself. Her behavior was preventing her from forming bonds with anyone in her life. I encouraged her to find positive male role models amongst her teachers, and even referred her to a male therapist who could serve as a male mentor for her and use transference techniques to help her learn how to develop healthy relationships with men.

Isabella also learned some of the techniques discussed in this book, such as meditation and emotional regulation, and although she maintained a preference for rough sex, she also learned to achieve pleasure and intimacy in sex rather than using it as a form of self-punishment.

Relationship 101: how to handle conflict

• • • •

I teach a lot of coping skills in my practice. One must learn how to handle conflict in productive ways. These are great skills not only to try in communicating with your child but also for them to use in communicating with each other, both in romantic relationships and beyond. These are key life skills, and play an extremely important part in the development of healthy intimacy at all ages.

Explain to teenagers that both passive and aggressive behaviors can result in issues. Being passive may sometimes seem like the safe option—but long-term passivity can lead to extreme resentment, and the relationship eventually becomes intolerable. In the short run, it might seem as though giving in will protect the relationship by avoiding conflict. But then the relationship takes a shape you can't stand in the long term. You'll start avoiding the other person or break it off. For example, if your friend takes you for granted and you never state the demands that would make you happy (attending your birthday party, for example, or calling you back), the relationship will come to feel one-sided, and eventually you may get super angry and explode, or, even worse, you might grow resentful and break off the relationship. Either way, this is not the road that leads to healthy communication.

Aggressive behavior also has its issues. If you feel you have been hurt or that someone has done you wrong, you may feel justified in acting out—blaming, screaming at, or threatening the other person. You may *think* you understand how other people should behave, but the reality is, it's very hard to see things from another person's point of view. Acting out will only alienate them further. You may also feel the need to punish them out of a sense of justice. This will inevitably result in you pushing people away. They will be scared to make themselves vulnerable to you or show you who they really are.

Either way, passivity and aggression both destroy relationships. The answer?

Assertive communication protects relationships... and I can teach you how

Assertiveness scripts are very important for getting your needs across in any relationship. Assertiveness protects both ends of the relationship and ensures that resentment and anger do not develop.

6 tips for assertive communication

1   Use *I* statements at all times. Avoid *you*!

2   *I think* (describe the situation): Stick to the facts, and use nonjudgmental statements about the facts.

    Example for teen: "I think that you told me you were going to hang out with me on Friday and not with your other friends."

    Example for parent: "I think I reminded you last week that we have a family night on Friday."

3   *I feel*: Use *I feel* statements ("I feel hurt/disappointed/frustrated"). And please stick to *I* statements at all times!

    Example for teen: "I feel hurt that you decided to cancel on me."

    Example for parent: "I feel frustrated that you are now asking to do something else when I was clear about what we were doing."

4   *I want*: Use *I want* statements to ask for exactly what you want. Do not assume others can read your mind, and do not place blame.

    Example for teen: "I want you to show up when you say you're going to."

    Example for parent: "This evening is important and I want you to cancel your plans."

5   Reinforce or reward the person ahead of time if they do what you like.

    Example for teen: "If you did not keep canceling, not only would it make me happy—but also, I would be able to rely on you."

Example for parent: "If you did cancel your other plans, it would make me happy and I would be willing to let you go out Saturday night and even give you some money."

6 Nonthreatening consequences (only if really necessary): This is telling the person what you will do if they keep up the same behavior. It's a gentle way of making it clear what the consequences will be without directly threatening.

Example for teen: "If you keep canceling on me, I will not keep the time set aside for you and will make other plans."

Example for parent: "If you are not able to attend the family night on Friday, then I will not be able to lend you the car for the rest of the week."

How to say no

When saying no, make sure you express empathy for the other person's perspective, and then clearly state your refusal. An example: "I can see why you want to go to John's party on Friday. It will be a lot of fun, but I cannot go as I have too much homework to do."

How to help your angry and irritable teen
• • • •

Help them change their expectations. Pinpoint what outcome they expected from an interaction or situation, and then what beliefs led them to expect such a result. Finally, brainstorm reasons that those beliefs might not be completely accurate. One might study hard for a test, for example, but still get a poor grade. That is a disappointing outcome, but it's no one's fault—neither theirs nor the teacher's—and getting angry doesn't change the result.

Help them communicate their expectations in relationships. Even the simple fact of vocalizing an expectation—"I don't think my boyfriend should talk to other girls"—can illuminate whether it is realistic or not. And if the expectation is unrealistic, help them understand the other person's perspective. Thoughts like "I expect my boyfriend to call me every night" might lead to anger when it doesn't happen, which will serve to polarize the other person, and drive them away or make them lash out in return.

Often, anger serves to protect self-esteem. If someone criticizes you or puts you down, you might get angry rather than feel sad. This is so you don't have to take accountability for your role in the situation. There is another option—you can admit responsibility but also preserve your self-esteem. The only person who can make you lose self-esteem is you, by allowing the criticism to speak to your own inner critic. For example, the teacher criticizes me, therefore he doesn't like me, or he thinks I'm stupid, or he's a lousy teacher. These are all examples of a maladaptive defense against losing self-esteem.

Dr. David Burns talks about anger and how it stems from people's ideas and concepts of fairness. Discuss this with your teen so they can learn to reflect on the bigger picture. It is easy to get angry when you perceive things to be unfair: my friends get a later curfew, or they all have iPhones and I don't, etc. Fairness is relative. It might be unfair that your parents give your younger sibling more attention, but if your sibling has a learning disability and has to work twice as hard to get the same grades, whose life is unfair, yours or your sibling's? In that scenario, the parents give extra attention for a good reason: the sibling needs the help. And it is also unfair that one sibling has to work harder to get the same grades. A teen might think it's unfair that the teacher makes her take off her hat at school, but from the teacher's perspective, they can't see the student's eyes and are not sure if she is paying attention or confused. Having a different perspective means seeing that the unfairness doesn't exist from the teacher's point of view; they're not doing anything to intentionally make your teen upset.

Dr. Burns believes that people get angry when they feel that things are unfair, but learning to identify and appreciate a variety of perspectives on an issue can deflect a negative, angry response. I like to challenge teenagers with this thought: is it better to be right or effective? It may be right to get angry when some injustice happens to you, but is it effective? Is the anger going to help you and the people you get angry at? Or is it going to cause more harm, polarization, and negative emotions for yourself and the people around you? If the latter is the case, then let the anger go, and increase your chances for one more moment of happiness.

Be your own bestie! Having a great relationship with yourself
• • • •

Psychological traits that are mentally healthy, like self-esteem, are developed over time, from your child's first steps to their graduation day. Mental health is not about preventing illness, but about promoting health. We give less thought to mental health than to other types of development, but children should be taught from their early years how to take care of their brains and their bodies. Your child should know that when you held them in your arms as a newborn, you weren't hoping they would turn out to be the "perfect" child. You were hoping they would be healthy, that they would dance, sing, and be happy. Imparting this image to them—that you wished them a beautiful life—is essential.

On the one hand, negative self-esteem can lead to depression, substance abuse, poor grades, eating disorders, and other issues. Negative self-esteem is also correlated with early-onset sexual activity and teenage pregnancy, as it affects how your child perceives their body and responds to peer pressure.

Positive self-esteem, on the other hand, affects our relationships with others—and ourselves—throughout the life course.

Healthy self-esteem is thus a critical ingredient in sex positivity—thereby strengthening one's ability to communicate with others, care for the self and body, set and maintain boundaries, and act in accordance with a set of values. Positive self-esteem reduces adolescents' likelihood of engaging in risky sexual behaviors, such as early sexual debut and multiple partners.

Self-esteem can have a protective effect when it comes to the potential negative effects of sexualization. In a 2013 *Body Image* study,

56 normal-weight college women were exposed to either three sexually objectifying music videos or three neutral music videos. Before and after the videos, the students indicated their perceived and ideal body size. Researchers found that women who had high self-esteem were not negatively affected by exposure to the videos. Women with low self-esteem, however, perceived themselves as bigger after watching the objectifying videos.

There are millions of pieces of information entering your mind even as you do something as simple as walk down the street. How this information is interpreted, however, is the key to living a healthy, happy, and productive life. Perception is the key to a healthy self-esteem.

Some professionals and parents worry that children can develop an inflated sense of self-esteem that prevents them from recognizing their own flaws and improving themselves. This is not a concern that I share, as I believe that a lack of self-esteem is a far more pressing issue. After all, there are many factors working against your child, especially when it comes to their burgeoning sexuality. Even healthy adolescents may experience fluctuations in self-esteem.

So, what can parents do to contribute to positive self-esteem?
• • • •

Explain media manipulation

Parents can resist media and social influences that encourage early sexualization. I do not see a need for a child to view fashion magazines, but if they do, thoughtful discussion should contextualize the images they see. Explain that the models are airbrushed or Photoshopped, for example. Some kids enjoy seeing the process of how an image is digitally altered, and there are many videos of this on YouTube that you can show them.

Similarly, some companies are now coming out against digital manipulation and engaging more realistic models. American Eagle launched a successful campaign called #AerieREAL, encouraging the use of an Instagram hashtag to show how their bathing suits and clothes look on real shoppers' bodies.

Keep the lines of communication open and actively discuss the pressure to achieve cultural ideals of attractiveness.

Continue to discuss and monitor social media as well, as many teenagers who develop eating disorders follow "pro-ana" or "thinspiration" discussion boards or blogs that feature social media icons who are dangerously skinny and give girls tips on how to obtain an unhealthy, anorexic body.

A recent study of middle and high school adolescents found that elevated "appearance exposure" when using Facebook—sharing photos on one's profile, viewing photos posted by friends, commenting on friends' photos, and tagging photos—was associated with a greater tendency to self-objectify and internalize a thin ideal, as well as weight dissatisfaction and a drive for thinness.

Importantly, it was not how much time overall was spent on Facebook that had a negative effect, but *how* that time was spent. In fact, social networking sites like Facebook can actually extend social support to individuals with low self-esteem and low life satisfaction, although strong offline social skills can make for a more beneficial online social networking experience overall. Parents can thus intervene to help adolescents improve their experiences online without forbidding the most popular contemporary forms of social connectivity.

Praise the right traits

Beginning in the early years, praise your child for their kindness, abilities, and strengths rather than their appearance. Use Disney as an example: the idea that the prince will save the princess is slowly changing, as evident in *Tangled*, *Frozen*, and *Moana*, where the females are not rescued but save everyone else. Still, sexualization in how the characters appear and what they wear has not changed much. Mattel has come out with a gender-neutral Barbie, where the hair can be changed and the doll is not leggy with breasts. This is a nice step forward, but only if boys are encouraged to play with it too.

Healthy role models can be chosen to show that value lies in what the body can do, not just in how it looks. Younger female athletes or other teenage role models who are of healthy weight can be referred to in discussions of body image or appearance. Continue to praise your teen for their efforts and abilities rather than their appearance. When trying on clothes for either yourself or your child, keep the focus on positive evaluations, such as strength, health, or unique features.

Appearance and presentation aren't everything

Preteens should be made to understand that school is not a fashion show, and that getting dressed quickly is a virtue, so their focus can be on learning.

As your child enters adolescence and then the teen years, it is important to realize that they will often struggle with accepting their body. Instead of just forbidding certain types of clothing, try to understand why your child is gravitating to a certain look. Does your kid only want to wear miniskirts that barely clear their underwear, for example? Maybe they are insecure about their growing breasts or some other mark of puberty, and want the focus to be on their legs. With boys, I have seen them start wearing big baseball caps to cover their hair and forehead to hide burgeoning acne, or to hide their eyes, as boys often get shy during early adolescence.

A Patient's Story: Lisa

MY PATIENT LISA told me a story about growing up in the South, where she was told by the matriarchs of her family that she needed to "put her face on" before leaving the house. This started at a very young age. Her great-grandmother would constantly "tut-tut" under her breath as she fussed with my friend's "too-large ears that stuck out" and tried to plaster them back with hairspray. She was also reminded throughout the day to suck in her stomach at all times. The message received was that her face wasn't good enough as it was and required painting to be acceptable for public consumption, and that she had to alter her diaphragm and breathing even if this interfered with her overall health.

So that's a great example of what not to do! Don't highlight a potential perceived flaw before your child has even thought of it. Kids will come up with enough on their own! But what *should* you do? If you continue to communicate about positive body image, minimizing any mention of their flaws, you can help them integrate the changes that they dislike with the parts of their body that they do feel comfortable with. One way you can do that: you may decide to allow the short skirts or a lower-cut blouse occasionally and when appropriate, because it helps them develop pride and confidence in their appearance. Better to allow it for certain occasions than to go out of your way making them feel nervous, uncomfortable, or shameful about their body. As a parent, you should empower your child to understand that appearance and presentation isn't all they are about. But letting them dress in a way that makes them feel beautiful and sexy can be empowering in the right settings, such as that school dance or prom, or in their free time during the weekends!

Another positive parenting moment related to appearance is allowing them to express some individuality. Let them have pink hair in the summer, let them experiment with their appearance. As long as it's not permanent, such as piercings or tattoos, giving them a little free rein will make them less likely to rebel too hard all at once.

Teach your kids about grooming practices. Shaving, deodorant, skin care, and other daily practices may seem like second nature to you, but it is surprising how many kids will forget even to brush their teeth in the morning! Good grooming will build self-esteem. I have had many children in the adolescent years, especially boys, who need very direct and strict rules around grooming, including demonstrations on how to shave or how to shampoo their hair, especially if they have social skills issues or ADHD. Sometimes you need to be a lot more direct in your instructions than you might realize as a parent. If they have acne, parents often need to buy them the appropriate products and show them how to use them. It can be shocking how little some teens care about their appearance. I have even had fathers of boys go into the shower with them and show them how to do everything, and stand outside the door three times a week to check that everything has been done right. On the one hand, it's a health issue, but on the other, you won't have many friends if you walk around with greasy hair and a pungent odor.

As for more cosmetic shaving, this is where things might get trickier. There is a difference between grooming you need to do for your health–"take a shower so you don't smell"–and what you need to do for your appearance. Most teen girls want to shave their legs and underarms because they have taken in cultural messages about body hair. Even many men "manscape," and therefore it is not just the girls who are shaving their bodies. In the seventies, it was fashionable for pubic hair to be full and thick; now, for most women, it is barely visible. The thought of my 13-year-old daughter taking a razor to her precious labia seems a little scary to me. As parents, we have to relax and realize that they will figure it out with some instruction. Let your children drive the bus in this area of cosmetic grooming; allow them to decide what they want and support them in their journey. As long as they are clean and their hair is combed and out of their face so it can be seen by teachers and society, then their personal preference must be respected so they develop a sense of what they want for their own body.

Teach bodily comportment. There are ways to sit, walk, and talk that reflect positively on a person at any age. These lessons don't have to be dogmatic, like "Cross your legs!" or "Look at me when I'm speaking to you!" Explain why it is more effective if you make eye contact when talking to someone: "it makes you seem more trustworthy," "it's easier for people to hear what you're saying," "it will make you appear more *attractive*." That last reason will grow increasingly motivating as your child becomes interested in dating. An open body posture, with shoulders back, makes you seem more confident and attractive.

Practice what you preach!

Your child has been observing your interactions with others since birth, and will notice discrepancies between your words and your actions by age eight. If you are concerned with promoting a healthy body image, teaching about gender equality, or encouraging your child to respect their body, be sure to practice what you preach. Watch any tendency to call yourself fat, talk about dieting, or denigrate your body, for example. Actions speak at least as loud as words. Praise your hips, your curves, and your unique features.

Recognize the connection between the irrational emotions of puberty and self-esteem

Of the teens that I see in my practice, many feel angry a great deal of the time. Although they cannot say why they have such intense feelings of anger, I usually connect it to trying to maintain their self-esteem. What I explain to parents is that the reason some teens are angry all the time is that they have raging hormones that fuel their adrenal cortical system, and this creates adrenaline surges. Teens don't understand WHY it is happening, so they create a reason for feeling what they are feeling. The brain is always trying to rationalize the world around it. When the cerebral cortex doesn't have a reason, it makes one up (and it is usually the parents, whom teens feel safest with and who are in the closest vicinity, who get the blame)!

There is a widely accepted theory in the study of cognitive neuroscience which explains that the cerebral cortex always tries to find deeper meaning than may actually exist. A simple hormonal influx could be too deeply interpreted by the cerebral cortex as it tries to create meaning; this can translate into BLAME in the minds of teens. So when your teen is sitting around in their room with raging hormones, they'll default to "emotional reasoning," which is a cognitive process whereby a person concludes that their emotional reaction proves that something is true, regardless of any observed evidence.

Plus, they are not used to the hormone surges the way we are as adults. A perfect example is PMS! Think about how you responded to PMS as a teenager compared with how you cope with it now, as an adult. Teens haven't learned the coping mechanisms that adults have figured out. We understand as adults that when we feel an emotion, it is not necessarily connected to an external event. We understand by adulthood that emotions can be connected quite simply to physiological processes inside us.

So now we get it with teens: raging hormones leads to trying to find meaning where there is none, which leads to emotional reasoning, which leads to blaming someone else and sending anger their way. Feeling angry at someone else means you don't see the role that *you* played in the situation. Shifting the blame outwards—projecting—protects against the loss of self-esteem that would occur if the person recognized their own contribution to the problem. Yet accepting blame, even partially, does not need to deflate your self-esteem. Beating yourself up over mistakes will do it, though! I try to work with teens to make them realize that people make mistakes, and that it is okay to do so—you acknowledge your error and then move on. The teenage years are a time of intense learning, so mistakes are unavoidable. But these years are also a good time to begin practicing what it means to "own" one's emotions, experience those emotions, and then let them go.

Of course, there are times when genuinely bad things happen, and a person has the right—even the *need*—to get angry. But most of the time we find ourselves in situations where anger is unnecessary and a waste of time. As Dr. David Burns, an MD and CBT (remember? The thought hole disruptor therapy!) expert, writes, a person cannot feel anger and joy simultaneously. Every moment spent angry, then, is a moment wasted. Dr. Burns also believes that anger results in, and derives from, unrealistic expectations. Beliefs such as "If I work hard, I will get a good grade," "If I have a boyfriend, he should call me every night," or "If I had real friends, they wouldn't leave me out of their plans" create unrealistic expectations that can make your teen feel slighted and angry.

Create rituals

A ritual is defined as a religious or solemn ceremony consisting of a series of actions performed according to a prescribed order. Rituals have been used throughout history. Why do people love rituals? Why are they so incredibly important to society? They've been used since the dawn of time to give people a sense of belonging and meaning. And those things are so fundamental to our self-esteem.

If you are a religious person, there are many rituals that are already embedded in your major life events and day-to-day practice. But if you are not particularly religious and/or you are the kind of person who wants to create your own custom-made family rituals, this can be an amazing way of developing your children's self-esteem, giving them a sense of purpose and belonging, a higher place, in your family's community.

Contemporary societies do not often use rituals to mark developmental milestones, except in some religious communities and sometimes in educational contexts (such as graduation). But rituals, even ones created within the family, can be a way to acknowledge and incorporate physical and emotional changes into the history of the family.

A company called Lunar Wild helps parents design a first menstrual cycle box filled with things for a girl's first menses, such as menstrual pads, candles, literature, jewelry, and a place for the parents to write inspiring letters to their daughter to commemorate the event. I love the idea of parents writing a letter to their daughter years before the event, about what being a woman means to them and their hopes and dreams for that child, and then giving it to her on the day of the first menses. It will build self-esteem, and help create a sex-positive adult who loves who they are and can embrace their body and sexuality.

It is much easier to find rituals for females than for males. In Hispanic cultures, a *quinceañera* celebrates a 15-year-old girl's dedication to home, faith, and family. The girl dresses up and has a large party. A debutante ball (cotillion) is a formal ball that includes the presentation of 16-to-18-year-old females to society, indicating their eligibility for dating. This is a mostly outdated tradition, but it continues in certain areas of the American South. There are also many examples of first menstrual ceremonies in African tribes.

But boys becoming men can also be something to talk about and celebrate!

Creating a gentle man
. . . .

We all hope our son will be the kind of man who will treat all women well at all times, from his mom to his sister and his dates... all the way to his future life partners. Many parents have taught their boys how to shake hands firmly, sit properly at the dinner table, and say thank you, yet so often we forget to teach sexual etiquette. It seems that the rise of the hookup culture has resulted in teens who will have sex without even sending so much as a text the next day, taking little ownership of the other person's resultant emotions, with the mindset of "I never promised them a relationship." When a boy becomes a man, it's important that he also become a gentle man. This should be your mandate.

Rituals can be useful in creating a healthy sense of self-esteem and can also help a teenager figure out his identity and his place within the community. There are many examples of celebratory rituals for boys who are entering manhood.

Among Native American cultures, there are ceremonies presided over by elders that center on a boy fasting alone at a sacred site used by many in the community for generations. During this time, the young person hopes to have a vision that will help him find his purpose in life and society. Dreams or visions may involve natural symbolism—animals or forces of nature—that requires interpretation by elders.

Within the practice of the bar mitzvah in the Jewish religion, before the boy reaches the bar mitzvah age of 13, his parents hold the responsibility for his actions. After this age, boys and girls bear their own responsibility for their actions and for upholding Jewish traditions, and are able to participate in all areas of Jewish community life.

The Boy Scouts have many coming-of-age ceremonies designed to uphold the values of the Boy Scout movement, all of which culminate in the obtention of Eagle Scout status. For this, a boy must gain the 21 merit badges required to demonstrate that he can live independently and is competent or excels in a variety of tasks.

A family is a tiny community unto itself, and parents have the possibility of creating unique familial rituals to induct their sons into manhood. The options for such a ceremony are limited only by your imagination. It's about your family, which is your tribe. Consider drawing up a list of tasks your son must learn to do independently. I think picking ones from different areas of life would be prudent. Below are some ideas to get you started.

Becoming a provider

Assess the boy's ability to earn enough money to buy something the family needs to contribute to the family's life, such as a new appliance, or to take the family to the movies. The object is to make a contribution that doesn't only serve his own needs.

Child rearing

Assess the boy's ability to spend a day babysitting a young child, cooking and providing for that child's needs, to gain experience in child rearing. Or start smaller, with taking care of the family dog without help.

Reproductive health education

Assign the teen some sexual health books to read, and then provide some quizzes and discussion at the end to ensure that the critical sexual education topics (such as the prevention of STIs) are understood. Great books such as *Girling Up* and *Boying Up* by Mayim Bialik and

Drawn to Sex: The Basics by Erika Moen and Matthew Nolan are good resources. Websites like amaze.org can also provide some helpful tools. Create a set list of online reading or assignments, to be followed by a quiz and discussion.

Discuss what it means to be an adult

Take the time to discuss adult responsibilities, such as the proper way to treat a woman, regardless of whether she is a mother, sister, friend, or potential girlfriend. Transitions are hard, and adolescence is painful at times; think about all the media messaging around the awkward experiences of puberty. All those painful coming-of-age stories—for example, *Juno*, *Diary of a Wimpy Kid*, and *The Wonder Years*—have taught us that this transition can be difficult. Creating positive rituals will ease the pain and remind your child that pleasures and delights also come with this transition.

Once you've chosen the tasks, decide how to mark the passage.

• • • • • • • • • •

A journey

To create the "separation" required of a rite of passage into manhood, consider sending your son on a service trip to a foreign country or on a journey guided by an organization like Outward Bound, to increase his independence and feelings of competence.

I love the idea of creating a ritual journey around a boy becoming an adult ready to take on adult responsibilities. Set out for a weekend celebration—perhaps a camping trip, or some other kind of adventure—to commemorate the occasion, inviting wise members of your community to take part.

Words of encouragement and guidance

It would also be great to commemorate the event with a book or a group of letters from family and community members in which they share their hopes and dreams for the child's future sexual life and the responsibilities and pleasures that await him. Even if family members cannot attend the ceremony, they can contribute in this way. Peers or older teens can be invited to write something about what it means to go from a boy to a man. This can be a useful tool for rereading throughout the boy's life.

A totem

Bequeath him a piece of jewelry such as a necklace or a memento with the date and a loving quote for him to keep with him. I know that it will become his most treasured item.

PUTTING TOGETHER any of these kinds of ceremonies around what it means to leave childhood might help make your son into the adult you need him to be.

Great relationships with the other humans of the world
• • • •

Now that we've provided some ideas on how to improve your child's relationship with themselves, let's talk about helping them maintain positive relationships with others. It is important for parents to help children navigate the relationships in their lives, whether it be with their peers or with romantic partners.

Friendship and love from ages 7 to 12
• • • •

It is not uncommon for children even in their early and middle school years to truly fall in love—not sexually, but romantically. We are hard-wired to experience bonding and attachment feelings well before sexual desire has kicked in.

I have seen children fall utterly and crazily "in love" with other children–speaking about them constantly, wanting to be with them, and jealously keeping them from forming other friendships. I have seen them absolutely heartbroken after the loss of a childhood friendship, to the point of serious depression and suicidal thoughts (even in a nine-year-old).

Many parents tend to minimize situations such as this, thinking it's not a big deal. When you minimize their feelings, you fail to validate your child's experience. The Dutch have embraced validation in their sexual education curriculum and in their society, feeling that children can indeed fall in love, in a way that is distinctly different from sexual attraction. It is common for grade school teachers to talk about crushes between classmates. Parent should do this as well, as it validates the heartbreak young children may feel when a relationship ends. That validation can help them grieve the loss, and these experiences provide great lessons for later in life, when they begin forming sexual relationships.

A Patient's Story: **Cailee**

CAILEE CAME TO me as a nine-year-old girl who had met the love of her young life, Sierra, at age six. They were neighbors and they did everything together—sleepovers, playdates, holidays. Cailee's older sister and Sierra's older brother began dating, and then Cailee's sister cheated on Sierra's brother. Sierra's brother then told Sierra she was no longer allowed to see Cailee. Sierra was told that the family was "bad news" and dishonest. Sierra abruptly broke off the friendship with some very fierce insults. Cailee was devastated, crying for days. Then Sierra found a new best friend and was often seen at school laughing behind Cailee's back.

Cailee came to me in a deep depression. She could not understand what had happened and how it all went so wrong, how other people in the class were not standing up for her. She thought about killing herself. She believed she would never have another friend. Every sad song trigged a flow of tears. She felt she would never be the same. Cailee's mom was not sympathetic, feeling she should just get over it and make some new friends. Cailee's mother tried to get Sierra to talk to Cailee and at least form some kind of relationship, but Sierra refused.

In treatment, I worked with Cailee to validate her experience and help her process the loss. Years later, at age 13, Cailee is still sad, and strangely enough, I feel much of it is over that childhood relationship. She really was in love, and the breakup caused her serious emotional damage.

I have seen teens try to commit suicide after a breakup. If they had had practice in the breakup of friendships when they were younger, and if they had had help from their teachers in navigating this, they would have been so much better off. It is important to reassure children that it is normal to fall in love with other children. Rest assured that it doesn't necessarily indicate the future sexual orientation of the child.

In middle school, social networks become even more important in the child's everyday life and can have an intense emotional impact. Your child may develop "crushes" or show increased interest in romantic situations. Some kids begin using social media and start to form tighter, more exclusionary groups. Differences between parenting styles may become more marked at this time, as some preteens are given a wide range of freedoms while others are more restricted personally and socially.

If you have a child who is in an intense relationship (in love) with another child, you might like to consider the following tips:

1   Validate the child's experience: "It seems you might have a real love for your friend."

2   Acknowledge the loss if this occurs: "Breakups happen. Even the loss of friendship can be hard."

3   Tell them emotions are like a wave: they will rise up, make a crest, and then go down. Grieving over a loss is normal and will get better over time. Sitting with the feeling for a while and crying it out will sometimes make it better. Distraction can also help. Time will certainly make the grief better.

Parents, embracing your child's feelings can validate their experience and help them navigate future relationships.

Curb the labeling

Kids may also start labeling others as "sluts" or "whores" based on their behavior or appearance, although girls are more likely to be on the receiving end of negative judgments. If you hear your child use the words "slut," "whore," "gay," or "faggot" as insults, correct them immediately. Ask them to imagine what it would be like to be "gay" and then to hear the word used negatively. Similarly, correct them if you hear the word "pussy" being used about someone who is acting fearful or cautious. Reaffirm that men can be feminine and kind, whether they are gay or straight. While you're at it, reaffirm that calling someone a slang term for a vulva is not rational, because vulvas are anything BUT weak!

Talking about how labels are used to connect sexuality and negative judgments about people will help your child avoid using slurs accidentally or purposefully. Using the word "slut," for example, is defining someone negatively based on their perceived sexuality rather than who they really are, and it is dangerous and unfair. Watch your own use of language as well. If your preteen says something or overhears you saying something like, "Do I look like a slut/ho/etc.?" realize that you are in the middle of a teaching moment. This would be a perfect time to correct yourself, or them, and say, "That's not what I should call a woman because of how she is dressed—even if that woman is me!"

Curb the bullying

Even healthy adolescents may crack under the pressure of bullying (or the pressure *to* bully). Youth who are incessantly teased or bullied exhibit more social and emotional problems, as well as poorer physical health.

If you suspect your child is being seriously bullied, try to reach out to the parent of the other child or to the school's psychological support services to intervene, as this can get very serious quickly. If it is not serious bullying and more like teasing, I think trying to normalize it is good. If it is about their sexuality (teasing about being gay or a "fag," for example), explain that they do not need to decide about their sexual orientation now, and try to normalize the diversity of sexual orientations by exposing them to appropriate role models of different sexual orientations (whether in the media or community members) to demonstrate that they can be happy no matter how they later define. In other words, they should be proud of who they may become no matter what and ignore the bully as he/she knows nothing about how awesome gay/transgender people are.

Depending on the type of bullying, you might try saying, "Everyone gets teased and the best thing to do is ignore it and focus on the people in your life who like and care about you." I like watching movies about bullies (such as *Wonder*) that show how kids persevere in order to reinforce the idea that they can be strong and overcome adversity. Growing to be extremely tall–six foot three–I got bullied all the time, from being called Stretch, to being laughed at ruthlessly for years after I banged my head on the ceiling while dancing at a party, to jokes of "How's the weather up there?" etc. I was so lucky that my father was always reinforcing the idea that it didn't matter because I was beautiful and tall, and that someday I would move on and it wouldn't bother me as much. I watched the movie *Tall Girl* on Netflix recently and had to laugh at what I saw. It reminded me of my own childhood, and watching it with my kids opened up a forum for a discussion about what happened to me and how I handled it. I told them that no matter what people say, it is only you who can cause yourself to lose self-esteem by taking it in, so stand tall.

Ramp up the proactive communication

These years are a time to increase communication rather than pull back. Conversations with adults about how one should be treated in a relationship are important and can have a positive impact on self-esteem. Providing your child with information and maintaining open communication is essential. Conversations with your preteen should involve active listening, not just lectures given by you, the parent. As children may develop some shyness during these years, you may find it useful to initiate a sensitive conversation during another activity that does not require eye contact, such as when you're driving the car or washing the dishes. Ask questions about the social media that interests them, about what their peers are talking about, and about what shows they are watching. If your relationship has been rooted in open conversations from the beginning, new topics and concerns will arise more easily than if you are just now attempting to broach them. But if you are just broaching them now, don't give up. The more you try, the more likely you are to develop open communication.

Bring up consent and respect at adolescence...

Sex is *not* a special realm where you can suddenly treat people poorly. Yet, for some reason, it seems the most basic courtesies are shed with each piece of clothing in a hookup. Perhaps this happens because sex is too often taught as something to hide away and be ashamed of, rather than as a realm of experience where your actions really matter. Or else sex is viewed as taking care of one's own needs, with everyone else being responsible for themselves. A sex-positive approach to consent brings the social aspect back into the picture.

Some parents argue that middle school is too early to begin having such discussions, but if sex is not presented as an activity detached from the rest of social life, then your conversations about sex don't need to stand out either. You can raise something as the opportunity arises. This might happen when you're talking about films or television shows, popular songs, your child's friendships, school interactions, social media, or countless other subjects. Trust me, not only will this help your child become comfortable enough to ask for help navigating the stickier issues that arise during adolescence—sexual and otherwise—but it will also be a lot easier on you than trying to impart your *values*, in addition to important facts, in a stiff, anxiety-ridden "Talk."

Teach the importance of being considerate

Teach your kid that if they are engaging in an activity with someone else, they should consider their partner's feelings—whether the activity is tennis, binge-watching Netflix, hooking up, or having sex. Remind them to consider whether a specific activity will be pleasurable for their partner.

Teach them to treat each partner respectfully, whether they expect to have a long-term relationship or not. Explain that if they notice that someone they wanted to hook up with seems drunk or high, they need to take care of that person rather than forging ahead with satisfying their own physical urges.

Inform them that bragging about their sexual exploits is poor form, just as bragging about their athletic ability or their family's income is poor form. It's crude and crass, and is not how to develop a healthy self-esteem.

Friendship and love in the teen years
• • • •

Boyfriends, girlfriends, breakups

Esther Perel, a therapist who studies adult love, states that love is an important experience in young adulthood, in part because it is temporary. Learning what it is like to love—and to endure heartbreak—gives one a base from which to form the next relationship.

Perel told me during a phone interview:

The most important thing your child can do at the end of high school and college is to fall in love. Hookups are not going to give it to you. This is how you learn about conflict and relationship heartbreak. You can take any course you want but nothing will be more important than this. It seems that teenagers are waiting until well into their 20s before they are even having a relationship. And so, they are lacking in creating their stories when it comes to intimate relationships. I don't see this when I go abroad [outside of the US]. In other countries, teens have relationships in their teenage years and parents are more accepting of this, and are more welcoming of the young partners into their family's life. Young adults learn both connection and rejection— not just loss and rejection. They learn the cycles of harmony, disharmony and repair that drive relationships—connection, disconnection, reconnection.

Perel inspires me to encourage parents to allow their children to fall in love and have the experience of rejection; they will learn valuable lessons while still under your careful watch. Parents, when you allow your children to love and process loss, you serve as a guide in creating the foundation of their happiness in relationships.

Sex-positive lessons from Tamera

If sex is prioritized for the sake of building self-esteem and building healthy relationships with others... what, really, could sex-positive parenting look like? Well, it *could* look, or at least be inspired by (for those less extreme!), something like Tamera.

The intentional community Tamera is an example of an out-of-the-box parenting structure. I heard about this community through the documentary *Monogamish*, by Tao Ruspoli, and was very curious about how they raise children. I was able to meet with two of the parents. Tamera is an "eco-village," located in Portugal, founded by a small group of individuals who wish to explore a variety of options for humans to live in harmony with themselves and the environment. As part of working towards an "ethical planetary culture," many of the permanent residents practice responsible nonmonogamy.

Tamera has started a "Love School," which they state works on the principles of truth in love, no deceit in relationships, no claims to possession (in relationships), and solidarity and mutual support. They raise children in an intentional community and have a school where children are educated about the values of Tamera (as well as receiving more traditional education). What I find really amazing about Tamera is their Parents' School. The Tamera website states,

> Raising and accompanying children in community isn't a private affair as the whole community takes responsibility for their care. Adults entering Tamera as parents or parents-to-be in the community must not see their children as "theirs" to privately possess, and must allow other people to have a say in how they raise them. This is the fundamental change from a private to a communitarian way of raising children, from fear to trust.

At the Parents' School, parents discuss questions about the children's position within the community and receive supportive feedback from the others. Facilitated by the leading team in their Children's School, parents and other caregivers raise consciousness about raising children.

I love the idea of parents getting together to discuss child rearing and helping each other through instruction but also through direct help with child care. Children don't come with instruction manuals, and I spend a lot of time in my practice on parent training. All the group therapy sessions I have started with multiple parents have been extremely popular, as parents feel validated by each other. I find Tamera's parenting school represents a utopian ideal–one that I wish could be more widely adopted in more mainstream schools.

To obtain a deeper understanding of their community, I interviewed several Tamerians by telephone.

A Human Story: Lyle and Katherine

LYLE AND KATHERINE are full-time "Tamerians" and parents. Lyle has an adult child from a previous relationship, and Lyle and Katherine also have two children together. The second of these children, a boy, was born within days of his half sibling, whom his father had conceived with another mother, named Dana. Lyle, Katherine, Dana, and the three children currently live together.

This kind of parenting arrangement is not unusual at Tamera. Tamera features many different types of parenting arrangements, and has a children's house where children can live separately from their parents for periods of time if they so choose. Parents are highly encouraged to attend the Parents' School, a kind of group therapy with elders of the community who are also parents. At Parents' School, the group discusses issues that arise across the child-rearing years, with a focus on helping children learn to be independent.

As Lyle explains, "Some of the things parents do actually make their kids become more dependent rather than fostering independence. We try to perceive our kids as big beings and souls that come to the earth, not just tiny cute people who need our help." When a toddler falls down and cries in mainstream communities, most parents rush to pick them, look for injuries, and comfort them. In Tamera, parents are taught to be conscious of how much their reaction will influence their child's experience. Parents will act undisturbed in such a situation unless there is a chance of real injury. Kids, then, often just pick themselves back up and continue playing. If a Tamerian adult sees a child sitting under a tree, either playing or just looking around, they will not approach the child and initiate conversation. Instead, children are given space, allowed to entertain themselves and let their thoughts roam. A child's need for privacy and immersion should be given precedence over an adult's desire for contact.

Sometimes, young children seek out breast milk from nursing mothers in the community who are not their own. Katherine says, "Children seek what they need from different parental figures. Sometimes my son needs me for nursing and sometimes he needs someone else. I try to be respectful of his wishes, and in the same fashion I allow him to get advice from others as well. His child rearing is very self-directed."

Tamerian parents also work to make the transition from adolescence to adulthood meaningful and enjoyable, sometimes borrowing from other cultures. Menstruation is not approached as a "curse" but as a personal milestone. When a girl gets her period, she decides who she wants to inform, whether friends or family. Girls may receive gifts from community members or, if desired, be at the center of a ceremony. Lyle's daughter wanted to go to the spring, which is a beautiful area of the community where many ceremonies are held, and invited important women in her life to conduct a ceremony for her, with a white dress and a horse. Other girls just want their mother involved. There is a lot of self-determination allowed for children in Tamera.

The first sexual experience is planned with an adolescent's parents and other mentors in the community. A young person may be in a relationship and feel they want to bond more intimately, or they may not be in a relationship but be curious to experience sex, or there may be other motivations they may choose to bring up. There is thought put into the expectation the couple has for the experience and for the future, similar to negotiating a mutually agreed-upon contract. There is no precise age for a first sexual experience at Tamera, but thought is put into whether the teen is mature enough to handle the experience. Most teens in the community are honored to ask and to be asked by one another, and show appropriate respect to the process. Consent is taken very seriously; the teens ask each other formally if they'd like to engage in this way. It's a more formalized process, not like American teens getting drunk at a party and hooking up without prior discussion. Another aspect of the experience is that appropriate birth control is obtained for the couple. Sometimes, friends of the couple gather together, the couple go off alone and have sex, and when they return, their friends welcome them back into the community.

Obviously, this represents a very different model from what's going on in mainstream American society. But in the Tamerian community's radical approach to openness around sexuality, there are some pearls of wisdom that even more vanilla parents can glean. The first is around the importance of acknowledging the transition between being a child and becoming an adult—the first menstrual period or, for a boy, the transition into manhood. The second pearl of wisdom is that there is merit to the idea of making sexual initiation something that is discussed and valued as important within the family. You should want your kids to consult with you on the topic and feel comfortable about sharing their fears and hopes around their sexual initiation. The third pearl is that the Parents' School provides a forum where they can discuss parenting ideas with each other for the betterment of the community.

Parents should not engage in ostrich syndrome. Burying your head in the sand does not mean your teen's sexual activity will not happen, and being part of the discussion does not mean you are pushing them into doing it. Rather, you are helping them to understand the risks and benefits. It's a great opportunity to be a part of their life and their decisions.

5

Sexual
Initiation

· · · ·

Sort out sex and romance by teaching rational love

• • • •

Many adolescents are told by their parents that it is best to wait until they are in love–or even married–to have sex. Certainly, there are parents for whom this sounds like good advice, while other parents remember that they did not wait and now they want to be more practical where their own children are concerned. It's important to understand the zeitgeist of your kids' experience, including the language they use to describe dating; most kids start using language that is very different from that of their parents. In my practice, I have never heard a teen use "dating" to describe what I would consider a romantic relationship. I have heard "talking to" and "hanging out," etc. So clarify what these things mean for your child so you can get on the same page.

Parents may differ on when a child should start dating, but regardless of your position, it is a good idea to discuss your beliefs with your child. Group activities make more sense during the middle school years, and explaining that "my parents won't allow me to date yet" can reduce peer pressure. Some older adolescents, however, are more interested in having fun than in commitment. Some are not emotionally mature enough to sustain commitments during these years; others may doubt that it is even possible. Teenagers are astute observers, and many have already learned that sex and love do not necessarily go together. This can be widely seen in the media, and

teens may also have witnessed parents or other adults changing partners or having sex without serious attachments.

What is the right age to begin having sex is a complicated question.
On average, the age of sexual debut has gone up, and currently sits
at around 16 to 17 years old. And teens are having sex less frequently
and with fewer partners than a few years ago.

We want our children to delay sexual initiation for as long as
they need to develop their minds and bodies. Research shows that
when parents express care for their kids with things like praise, hugs,
and careful sharing of values, there is a positive delay in sexual initiation as well as other healthy outcomes. Parental control is also
linked to these positive outcomes, but this is a more complicated
subject. If parents are exercising control by monitoring their children's whereabouts, or using things like curfews, this can result in
delayed sexual initiation. But if parents are controlling by trying to
limit who their children may interact with and how often they can
date, this over-monitoring can often result in a backlash, with dating
disagreements (tiger parents beware) and sneakier and noncompliant
behavior, and early sexual initiation.

The Guttmacher Institute, which does sex research, informs us
that the teen pregnancy rate has dropped to a third of what it was
in 1990. At first blush this sounds like a good thing, but it has come
at a cost: teens are now living in a virtual world, interacting on their
phones and not in real life (and this makes physical sex impossible).
And they're not hanging out, lazing around, and connecting (sexually
or otherwise); instead, they are getting lonely, sad, and more anxious.
This has resulted in the teen suicide rate going up since 2000, with
sharp increases in the last four years—and it is not only the kids who
are affected by the lack of sexual behavior. The *Atlantic* published an
article about how we are entering into a sex recession, where sex is
happening more online than in person. Adults too are having sex less
frequently, according to the results from the General Social Survey
by the independent research organization NORC. The average rate
of sexual activity went from 62 to 54 times a year (from over once
a week to under) between the 1990s and 2014. Some explanations

for this decline include lack of coupling, coupling later in life, lack of cohabiting with partner, sleep deprivation, anxiety, antidepressant use, and the rise of online pornography.

We want our children to have sex when they are ready and emotionally capable of handling it, but we don't want them to wait until they're older only because of lack of free time, eternal stress, and access to free-flowing porn, as all of these things come at a price as well. The cost is an inability to form intimate and healthy relationships, which by every measure of psychological well-being are a key predictor of happiness. There is a balance that needs to be struck between waiting to be mature enough and embracing your sexuality when you're ready. The sexual relationship practice that you get in your late teens and early adult years is critical to the development of the skills needed to foster long-term bonds before you have the pressure of raising children or other serious responsibilities.

It can be difficult to figure out exactly the right message to send about sexual and romantic relationships. Should parents continue to at least *try* to get their teens to wait for such a relationship? Or should we revise our expectations to fit a contemporary world? A world where we do not even necessarily want our children to fall in love during the teenage years, much less marry that first boyfriend or girlfriend and never date again?

Acknowledging that there are many reasons to have sex, from showing commitment to wanting to be liked, from a desire for pleasure to simple curiosity, may help your teen decide what matters to *them*. One great way you can help your teen navigate this for themselves is by explaining the concept of "rational love."

Rational love is a philosophical approach to relationships focused on sharing a relationship that is based on intimacy, trust, and mutual respect. This precept can be applied regardless of whether a sexual relationship is long- or short-term. Rational love means that love is based on some amount of reason and intellect rather than just instinct, intuition, and romance.

Flirting training

• • • •

The definition of "flirt" is "to behave as though attracted to or try-ing to attract someone, but for amusement rather than with serious intentions." When sexual initiation begins, it is very important for teenagers to understand the importance of flirting and rejection prac-tice. Many of the teens I work with may have social skills deficits, such as mild autism, and may be a bit behind socially. Some have ADHD and are socially immature, while others are just shy. These teens are often frustrated that they cannot find a boyfriend or girlfriend (or even just get a date to the school dance). They may feel rejected and have self-esteem issues. Parents, this is where flirting training comes in handy. And you can help teach these important social skills to your child. Flirting is the first step towards sexual initiation, and it is an important part of dating. But you do not need to be sexually attracted to someone to flirt, or have the intention of dating them. Flirting is just a skill that can be practiced and used in all aspects of life. You can flirt with almost anyone as long as you keep it platonic–but you can also flirt with someone you might be interested in dating, as this is the first step in many along the road to intimacy.

4 steps to flirting

1   Make the other person feel special and admired. Praise anything you can; try to get them to talk by asking probing questions.

2   Smile, and hold their gaze a little longer than you would normally.

3   Tease the other person in a friendly way, as you would with a fam-ily member you like. (Don't be mean or overly negative, though.) Laugh at any jokes they make.

4   Use positive body language. Get closer to them (if they seem com-fortable), and maybe just touch their arm (if they seem receptive).

Get rejected

• • • •

Once you have embraced flirting and are ready to ask someone out, then you have to get ready to be rejected. This is also an important part of dating, and an important part of life in general. How you handle rejection will have an immense impact on your happiness.

Asking someone to go on a date means making yourself vulnerable, and this takes courage. This is the foundation of researcher Brené Brown's work on the subject. Part of being vulnerable is allowing yourself to get rejected. This is the opposite of avoidance. Avoidance is based in fear—fear of rejection—and this fear is always fooling yourself, because if you avoid going after what you want, you will never get rejected, but you also will never experience success. Brown states that fear will always be there to greet us, as it is a restrictive force that stops us from stepping outside our comfort zone towards the realization of our true desires. But fear can be conquered, because in this case fear of rejection exists only in our mind. If we do get rejected, we will be no worse off than we were before.

Dr. Albert Ellis, one of the founders of CBT, was famously shy. It is said that he challenged himself to speak to 100 women at the Bronx Botanical Gardens, with the intention of finding a date, to overcome his fear of rejection. In the process he learned that rejection was not as bad as he had feared. He then went on to become a famous CBT expert and even a famous sexologist, with awesome advice on love and dating.

What I have learned from Dr. Ellis is that rejection is a vital part of life—and when you are looking for love and intimacy, rejection will be part of the process. Being able to bounce back from rejection is critical to finding intimate relationships. If you avoid taking a chance for fear of getting hurt, then "nothing ventured nothing gained," and you will be alone.

Jason Silva, a TV personality and a philosopher, talks about rejection in a video on his Instagram page called "Have You Ever Been Rejected?" He states, "Agony and ecstasy are two sides of the same coin; without the bitter, baby, the sweet is not as sweet. When the ones we love tell us 'no way,' we take it in and we accept it with grace and we feel the ache in gratitude." Parents, you can teach this to your children. Rejection is good; it is practice for what will happen all the time in life. Teach them not to be afraid to try, to ask that person out, even if it is just for a study group, and if they get rejected, then they should not take it to heart. Chances are the other person will be flattered and be even kinder to them in the future. Many of us remember that person who asked us out and whom we turned down—and whom we were always kinder to afterwards.

A Patient's Story: Owen

OWEN IS A 16-YEAR-OLD boy with mild autism, which used to be known as Asperger's. When I first met him, he was socially immature and introverted. Yet he is a tall and great-looking boy; he is a good student who also attends robotics club, where he is well-liked. He came to me because he felt he didn't fit in. He did have friends but had a hard time speaking to the opposite sex. He could not understand what it would take to find a girlfriend. In therapy, we discussed combination skills and began the process of flirting training and rejection practice (both described above). He practiced on many people that he met and understood that getting rejected does not leave you any worse off than if you just avoided people in general. Either way, you end up with no dates. And he learned that even when he asked a girl out and she was not interested, she was usually nicer to him in the hallways after—whether out of sympathy or from a feeling of flattery at having been asked. For whatever reason, the girls paid him more attention afterwards.

We talked about how self-esteem comes from your views about yourself, and how only you can cause yourself to lose self-esteem. Owen used this to his advantage, telling people right away that he was shy and sometimes awkward. He disarmed them with his vulnerability, and he started to work on the cardinal features of flirting—practicing them at school, after school, with his sister's friends at home, and then reporting back to me. I watched a Netflix show called *Atypical* that reminded me of these sessions, and I had to laugh at the father/therapist's involvement in the process of the son learning how to flirt. For my Owen and the character in *Atypical*, flattery, gentle teasing, and making good eye contact were skills he practiced, along with asking probing questions and moving closer to the other person. I even had Owen practice on his mom when he wanted to get some money out of her for a computer game he wanted. This resulted in great progress, and within a year he had a prom date. He met a girl who shared his interest in anime. He began dating and even had his first kiss.

What he and I both learned is that you can't take these basic social skills for granted, and some kids need a little more help to learn things that may be obvious to others. Parents, you can play a role in laying this foundation.

The evolution and neurobiology of sex— and how it pertains to your kids...
• • • •

Hormones and teenagers

Teenagers are often said to be thrown off balance by their "raging hormones." But what exactly does that mean?

In many ways, we are each a product of our brain. Many of our behaviors have been reinforced for evolutionary fitness through thousands of years by a combination of genes, hormones, and neurotransmitters, and understanding these aspects of development will make parenting easier.

Let's look at the basics of biology that are making your sweet child into an eye-rolling teenager.

Testosterone: A hormone that causes more masculinization of the male body but is also found in women. Masculine traits include increasing muscle size and mass, enlarging of the Adam's apple with deepening of the voice, increased secretion of oil and sweat glands (often causing acne in teens), and lower body fat percentage. Testosterone is also involved in increasing aggression and sex drive (but not affection) in both males and females. It can also promote traits that are traditionally thought of as "male," such as visuospatial ability and violent behavior.

Luteinizing hormone: Triggers ovulation in females.

Prolactin: A mostly female hormone involved in the menstrual cycle and milk production.

Estrogen: A hormone causing more feminization of the female body, including enlargement of the breasts, widening of the hips, and the accumulation of more subcutaneous fat than in males. Estrogen is also involved in the regulation of the menstrual cycle. It promotes sexual behavior in females as well as a sense of well-being and neuronal growth and cognition (in the earliest part of the cycle, when it is highest).

Oxytocin: A hormone involved in social bonding. It is released in both males and females during sex, and ensures closeness and attachment, i.e., "nesting behaviors." It is also released during milk letdown in women who nurse, and helps promote attachment between mothers and babies. In men, oxytocin is five times higher during sex and immediately drops after intercourse. It stays around longer in females (which may explain why some men want less cuddle time than women).

Vasopressin: Involved in regulating the amount of water absorbed in the body—and may be involved in water retention and high blood pressure. But it also plays a role in sexual activity, and is released in men during the arousal phase to help with erection and causes an increase in motivation to engage in sex. It can also promote aggression, and engenders paternal behavior by bonding males towards partners and offspring. Vasopressin is related to feelings of possessiveness and jealousy, and can promote competition between males. (It is also known as the jealousy hormone.)

Dopamine: The neurotransmitter that plays a major role in rewarding behavior. If it feels good, then dopamine was involved.

Serotonin: A neurotransmitter involved in many areas of the brain, and also in the GI system to regulate digestion. A simple explanation of serotonin's influence is that higher amounts mean less anxiety and depression.

Teenagers' hormone levels aren't technically higher than those of adults, but because they have not become accustomed to the effects of sex hormones, they are particularly susceptible to their influence. Testosterone, estrogen, and progesterone are all present in the bodies of children, but the levels rise significantly during adolescence, triggering physical changes.

Why is my teen girl moody? One minute she's fine, the next she's crying

Moodiness can be associated with the menstrual cycle due to hormonal fluctuations. Early in the cycle, the adolescent female's brain is dominated by estrogen. During this period, a woman may feel happy, peaceful, and even more social than usual, as estrogen can dampen the effects of adrenaline and other stress hormones. On day 14, luteinizing hormone surges to induce ovulation.

The release of the egg then triggers an increase in progesterone, which prepares the body for the implantation of a fertilized embryo by thickening the lining of the uterus. This phase also brings more emotional changes. The premenstrual phase makes some women feel tired, irritable, anxious, absentminded, and even unmotivated; other women barely notice these changes. Some women also experience physical effects such as tender breasts or food cravings that are related to these rapidly shifting hormone levels.

Adult women grow accustomed to these effects, and may be able to identify the day their period is starting by such changes in their emotional state. You can help your daughter by suggesting that she track her cycles on a calendar or app, and make note of her mood throughout the month. The first year or so of menstruation can be unpredictable—some girls menstruate every month, but others do so only a few times a year—but paying attention to hormonal fluctuations and how they potentially affect one's mood, sense of physical well-being, productivity, decision-making, and other things can be very useful. For girls who experience severe mood swings, hormonal birth control may bring some relief.

The teenage brain and risk taking

Magnetic resonance imaging (MRI) studies have taught us that adolescent brains are not fully mature. Although the neurons are mostly already in place at birth, the connections between the neurons and the myelination—the fat surrounding the neurons that conducts electrical impulses—are not complete. In other words, the roads are mapped out, but the paving has not been completed. According to Frances Jensen, author of *The Teenage Brain* and a neurologist, this means that your teen's brain is 80 percent connected and mature when it comes to things like verbal skills or muscle coordination, but they still might have difficulty thinking about the repercussions of their actions a few steps down the line. That 20 percent of the brain that is still developing could be blamed for some of the mood swings, impulsiveness, inability to focus, and risky behavior associated with adolescence.

Another reason that your teen might take risks which seem unnecessary from an adult's standpoint is simply a lack of experience. Jensen writes,

> Risk taking offers neurological rewards. When you take a risk there is a surge from the adrenal glands and dopamine is released into the nucleus accumbens which means we get instant brain high. But then if consequences ensue for bad choices we suffer later from the down side, the anxiety, and remorse, depression

and the brain low. Teens haven't experienced many of the consequences of their behavior and don't have the bad memories of it
to caution their decisions. As we make dumb decisions, however,
the memory of the negative repercussions that we experience (or
that we realize we could have experienced) dampens our enthu-
siasm for taking certain types of risks. For a teenager who hasn't
experienced negative repercussions yet, the anticipation of a
reward and achieving that natural high can be all he/she needs
to press forward.

When talking with a teenager about risk taking, it can help to ask
them to visualize the outcomes of their behavior rather than simply
giving a warning. "Use a condom so you don't get pregnant," for example, may be less powerful than having an adolescent girl imagine what
it would be like to walk into school with all her peers knowing she was
pregnant. Dr. Jess Shatkin, a mentor and colleague of mine at NYU Lan-
gone Child Study Center, writes in his book *Born to Be Wild* about the
process of attaching the emotion to the facts. For pregnancy, he writes:

> Adolescents generally try to avoid this discussion, but I'm relent-
> less. And as we walk painstakingly through each step of what
> happens next (e.g., "How do you tell your parents? Do you have
> the baby or get an abortion? What do you say to your friends? Do
> you graduate on time? What happens to the gymnastics team?"
> etc.), a light always goes on in their heads. The emotional feeling,
> not just the abstract thought, of what it would be like to actually
> get pregnant starts to sink in. This technique can counter an
> adolescent's sense of ambiguity or uncertainty about the pos-
> sible outcomes of a risky behavior, and I find kids to be much
> more realistic and grounded about their choices after this sort
> of conversation.

However, no matter what you say, teens will take risks, as they
generally think they know better and that bad outcomes and consequences won't happen to them. So the best course of action for all
parents is to make the good choices easy (buy them things they want

in return for good grades or getting home on time) and make the bad choices hard (grounding them, cutting off phone access for risky behaviors). This is a parenting language all teens can understand.

Explain emotional and physiological effects of sex
• • • •

Teens also need to understand the emotional and neurochemical effects of sex. When you have sex with the same person repeatedly, you become neurochemically bonded to them through oxytocin. This bonding process is important to humans as a species, because it makes reproduction more successful. Parents who are bonded together are more likely to help each other raise their offspring during the most vulnerable phase of development, whether that is for one breeding season, as is the case with king penguins, or for several years, for example with humans. Oxytocin is joined by vasopressin, a hormone that influences feelings of possessiveness and jealousy, and serotonin, a neurotransmitter that can fuel the more obsessive aspects of romantic love. Sex also stimulates the dopamine or "reward" system in our brain, which motivates us to pursue sex as a species and rewards us for doing so with pleasurable feelings. Dopamine levels in the brain increase during adolescence, and therefore adolescents are more likely to risk more for the sake of a higher reward, with less understanding of risks due to a lack of life experience.

Even "casual" sex serves up a potent chemical cocktail, with natural, but potentially unsettling, effects. The downside to the intense bonding that can accompany sexual activity is that it is all too easy to become bonded to a partner who is not suited to be part of your life long-term. Teens can also become emotionally overwhelmed by intense feelings of desire that create a roller-coaster experience ranging from the ecstasy of being in love to crushing heartbreak when the relationship ends. I have seen teens who were unprepared for such intensity, and who developed obsessional thinking and serious depression that manifested in self-esteem crises, self-injury, and even suicide attempts. Others may continually seek new relationships, avoiding the strong feelings of attachment and instead chasing the more immediate "high" of sexual activity.

Understanding the underlying biological processes that occur when we become intimate with someone can help teens (and their parents) make more knowledgeable decisions. After all, even adults can become swept up in the elation accompanying a new intimate relationship. Explain to your child that the emotional mind is impacted by hormones, evolution, biology, and cultural influences, and that it may be telling us to do things that jeopardize our ultimate well-being, but that our wise mind can use information from our emotions and our reason to create a balance. Rational love can be taught and brought up repeatedly through the years as a way to bring reason and intellect back into the picture. Rational love also provides a clear ethical stance from which to interact with both current and previous partners. Teach your child the utmost importance of treating each partner with kindness and respect, regardless of the outcome of the relationship.

The message here is that even with the hormone highs of a new romance, it's important to remind your teenager that this might not be the be-all and end-all, to keep a level head, and to remember that life is long! After a breakup, when all that dopamine from the sex wears off, help your child to remember that the person they were with is not their enemy. It's important to remind your teen to frame failed relationships as lessons learned in preparation for the next relationship–that is the energy they should be channeling.

Under pressure
• • • •

At the same time as teens are hearing about all this love and hormone stuff, they also face intense pressure from peers to engage in sexual activity. A teen girl may be led to feel guilty about saying no, or may worry that her boyfriend will break up with her if she does not have sex. A teen boy may believe that he should be having sex to prove his masculinity or heterosexuality, regardless of whether he is attracted to, or even likes, the girl. Both sexes may worry about being ridiculed for retaining their virginity.

The desire to maintain a relationship can be very strong for teens. A healthy sense of self-esteem can help buffer the threat of losing a boyfriend or girlfriend over sex. This underlying self-esteem might still need to be coupled with both an understanding that they are likely to eventually face a situation where they feel pressured and knowledge of *how* to assert themselves when necessary.

Parents can rehearse scenarios with teens, helping them devise comfortable ways to resist peer pressure. Reinforce the idea that sex is best in a trusting, caring relationship. If this is an ongoing discussion, your teen will already have a foundation from which to make decisions: *Do I want to have drunk sex, and be ashamed in the morning? Do I want to have sex with someone who might not even talk to me tomorrow? Should I share my body with someone whom I otherwise wouldn't even want to spend time with?* You can assure them of this:

Bad sex is not better than no sex at all. In fact, good sex is worth the wait.

• • • • • • • • • • • • • • • • •

Remind your teen that it is never too late to say no—even if it is the eleventh hour, the boy bought you lobster for dinner, or the girl is standing in front of you naked.

Teach your teen how to recognize the signs of manipulation or peer pressure from a partner: offering to be a boyfriend or girlfriend in exchange for sexual activity; saying "if you loved me, you would do it"; threatening to break up or to tell others about what happened; agreeing to stop, but only stopping the behavior momentarily or continuing to press boundaries in other ways; using put-downs or slurs as punishment; requesting that no one else be told; claiming that some activities, such as fellatio, are not really "sex"; and so on.

Practice responses to specific potential manipulations. For example, your teen can respond to "if you loved me, you'd do it" with a statement that shifts responsibility, such as "if you really loved me, you wouldn't try to make me do something that I don't want to do." For teen girls, bringing up having their period usually works quickly to dissuade an over-eager partner; boys could claim to be too tired or that they are expected to perform athletically later or the next day. Suggesting another activity, or suddenly noticing that it's time to get home, are other possible escape tactics.

Help your teen resist guilt, fear, or other negative emotions stemming from their decision not to have sex. Tell them that you think it's cool that they're waiting, and that you are proud of their decision. Remind them that the longer they wait, the more likely it is that the sex they have will be fun and meaningful, as they will be more mature and will know more about what they want. There are many studies to back this up—such as that teens who have earlier sexual initiation are more likely to have depression and suicide risk, and that teens girls who engage in oral sex at a younger age are less likely to be satisfied in their relationships later. Encourage discussion as to the pros and cons of waiting.

The pressure to have sex is real and intense. Educate your teen on the creative ways that girls and boys manipulate each other into doing things they don't want to do (and of course it's a manipulation!). Help them not to fall for it. You and your teen can practice saying out loud the things I've listed in the "top comebacks" section (below) and have a good laugh.

Top comebacks your teen can use to get out of a situation where they don't want to have sex

Says that if you loved them you would do it.

> "If you really loved me, you wouldn't try to make me do anything that I don't want to do."

> "I love you, but I am just not ready."

Says they'll break up with you if you don't give them what they need.

> "Well, that would be sad for us both, but much better than having sex and *then* breaking up. That would just be super-awkward."

> "Let me just clarify. Are you saying that if I don't have sex with you, then you'll break up with me?" (wait for response)

Tells you that you got them aroused and they'll get blue balls if you don't finish.

> "Your penis will be just fine. It's not like this is the first hard-on you've gotten that didn't end in sex."

> "You can't force me by making me feel bad. I still don't want to do it."

> "I know you can take care of this yourself after I leave!"

Agrees to stop, but then keeps trying in other ways, for example stops touching your breasts but then begins kissing your mouth, and moves again to kissing your breasts three minutes later.

> "I already said no to this. Perhaps it's best we stop kissing and watch a movie."

> "Hey handsy, are you the kind of guy who can't take no for an answer?"

Offers to be your boyfriend or girlfriend if you agree to sex.

> "Well, let's try out being boyfriend/girlfriend first, then we can decide to have sex later."

Says that they won't enjoy sex if they have to wear a condom.

> "No glove, no love."

> "I think condoms are super-hot, can I put it on you?"

Says that they won't "cum" or "ejaculate" inside you so you won't get pregnant.

> "We still need to get a condom, haven't you heard of pre-cum?"

> "Hey, I'm worried I'm so sexy you may not be able to control yourself, so we better find some condoms."

Says that things besides intercourse (like oral sex) aren't real sex, so they don't count.

> "Sex or not, I don't want to put your penis in my mouth."

> "Listen, let's just take it slow. Let's make out, then go and get pizza or watch a movie."

Says you're not a real man if you don't take her down.

> "Listen, man, I don't kiss and tell."

> "I don't need to brag about my sex life."

Calls you a prude and threatens to tell others.

> "That's so immature to threaten to spread rumors about me."

> "Do you think threatening to gossip about me will make me want to have sex with you? Try flattery and kindness first."

Makes false promises to not tell anyone, or threatens to tell people you're still a virgin.

> "It's not about saving my reputation, it's that I am just not ready."

Useful in any situation

> (For girls) "I think I just started my period and need to get some tampons."
>
> "I gotta get home, my parents are going to kill me!"
>
> "I don't feel comfortable, so I'm going to leave, but maybe we can talk later."

Hookups! Etiquette! Anal! Address the awkward
• • • •

So those are ways you can help your kid stay out of sex when they aren't ready. But when your teen starts to have sex, I'm here to tell you that it's totally appropriate to acknowledge the topics your parents never acknowledged with you–things like hookup culture, sexual etiquette, sex in the home, and anal sexually transmitted infections. Here are my thoughts on these.

Hookup culture is a thing, and you need to address it

Humans have evolved to feel intense love in intimate relationships, which develop through repeated episodes of sexual intercourse. Yet in my work with adolescents and college coeds, I have seen firsthand how young people are disconnecting from the intimate and sensitive feelings they have while having sex by getting drunk, thereby numbing the emotions that might engender feelings of love and connection. They are overriding that natural attachment impulse through the use of alcohol or by subscribing to the repeated cultural messaging that says it's better not to get attached. That "friends with benefits" messaging creates a sexual climate where young people are having less-frequent sex with more partners... which is often less fulfilling. So many articles are being written now that reinforce all of this. There's even a trend where young men are encouraged to hook up drunk, and then not to see those women or have sex with them sober. It also seems, from my own work with teens, that many college women are allowing men to dictate how the relationship will proceed.

A Patient's Story: Gracey

ONE OF MY CLIENTS whose story reflects the difficulties of hookup culture was a college coed named Gracey. She was raised in a sex-positive environment, and her mother, father, and brothers always supported her and encouraged her to have relationships based on love and trust. She left for college feeling very good about her body and her sexual needs, but soon found the culture to be different than she expected. No one dated, and most sexual encounters occurred while drunk. There was no texting each other the next day. Even though she wanted to have sex and the experiences she had were consensual, she rarely had an orgasm or experienced real pleasure.

On her birthday, she ran into a guy she found very attractive. They were drinking that night, they had sex, and because of their "good chemistry," she had an orgasm. She woke up happy and wanting to spend time with him in bed, but she felt the pressure to leave the room and avoid being needy. When he didn't text her the next day, she was upset but not surprised. She wondered how she had lost control of her emotions, and why she was afraid to reach out to him for fear of seeming crazy or overbearing.

Gracey felt sad. It was so rare for anyone in her college to have a boyfriend or to feel that the sexual encounters they were having were sexually pleasurable and fulfilling.

We spoke about how, even if she can't change other people's behavior, she can change her own, and that she might consider bringing a guy back to her room and saying, "Hey, you know, I want you sexually, but let's take a break here and meet again when we're sober." And if she did decide to have sex, she could reach out to the person the next day and say, "Hi, I really enjoyed what happened last night." If they don't write back, add: "I feel hurt that you didn't write back after we shared that experience together."

So, how can we encourage our kids to understand and work with this reality? We can start by educating them on realizing and accepting that although a sexual partner may be temporary, the experience can be both temporary and also kind, loving, and connected; these qualities don't need to be mutually exclusive. Temporary is okay, but basic sexual etiquette should be demanded and expected.

For some ideas on how to instill sexual etiquette and "gentleman/gentlewoman/gentle human" behavior, see the following sidebar.

Basic sexual etiquette for the sexually active

- Sex will be less fulfilling when you're drunk. Wait a bit to sober up—talk, hang out, quit the alcohol, and then you can really experience the fun and joy in sex.

- Make sure to ask your partner what he or she likes sexually—don't be afraid of pillow talk!

- It can be tricky to speak too much about past sexual experiences with new sexual partners. Although it is tempting to share all the details of your past life with someone new, it might be better to wait until you have developed real trust and friendship, especially when one partner is more experienced than the other. It is a good idea to explain and teach your partner that although you may have had experiences in the past, *this* is the experience you want to focus on now, and that "speaking out about past experiences won't help us live in the moment."

- Even if the relationship is not going to last forever, it's okay to love *in the moment*. Compliment your partner, tell them what you like about the way they smell, feel, and look. Not only is it kind, but it will turn your partner on and make the experience better.

- Call the other person the next day, even if it's to say that you don't think you can be in a relationship with them. Tell them that you wanted them to know how much you enjoyed the evening. This will avoid hard feelings on both sides.

How should you handle your teenager having sex in the home?

I believe that teenagers have safer sex in their own home than in a car or at a party, where other teens might be drinking and there is no possibility of you monitoring their behavior. If you are having an allergic reaction while reading this, consider the alternatives: having sex in public, in a bathroom, or even in a car could be illegal. I would hate to see a wonderful teen get arrested for public displays of nudity or lewd behavior while having sex. Teens should be informed of those legal risks.

However uncomfortable this may seem, keeping teens safe by keeping them in the home is the best option. If you know that your teen is having sex in the home, it is appropriate to go over the rules of your household—just as you would go over the rules for other situations—with your teen and their partner. Teens should be respectful of other family members, and not engage in any sexual behavior in front of siblings. The door to the bedroom should be closed and locked, and they should be careful not to make noise. Putting on some music is a great way to be discreet and respectful of other family members.

I also believe it is important to remind your teen that they are part of a family, not just a couple. Having sex isn't a reason to miss dinner, not do chores, or fall behind on schoolwork. The partner should greet other family members, not sneak away into the bedroom. If you are asking, "Is it really appropriate to lay down the rules and discuss sex with your teen's boyfriend or girlfriend?" the answer is yes, although boundaries are necessary. Try to get to know his or her parents, so that there are open lines of communication and you all know what is going on. Some families might be comfortable discussing ground rules together. Other families may disagree about what teens should be allowed to do in their bedrooms or home. Even if you do not agree with the other parents, it is beneficial to attempt communication. The same goes with same-sex relationships.

Handling STIs!

You can offer to buy condoms, and provide resources on healthy, safe sex (anal or otherwise). Any sexually active individuals should be tested regularly for STIs. Young women will possibly be tested during their annual gynecological exam, but young men may need to request tests at regular doctor's visits. If your teen encounters a negative outcome with an STI test and needs to share the information with one or multiple sex partners, it's beneficial to help them move past blame and handle these infections the way we'd handle strep throat.

Handling ANAL!

Both LGBTQ+ and straight teens may consider having anal sex, so it is appropriate for a parent to address this topic if desired. Even *Teen Vogue* featured an article, "Anal Sex: Safety, How Tos, Tips, and More," to address this issue in the mainstream, and it is a great resource to share. Parents can explain that anal sex can be very pleasurable. Some people with vaginas are able to experience orgasm from anal sex because their anus is close to the vaginal wall and pelvic floor, which means anal sex can stimulate the clitoris from the inside. Most people with penises have a pleasure point called the prostate inside the anal canal that can lead to an orgasm when massaged. In other words, pleasure through the back door is possible no matter one's gender, gender identity, or sexual orientation. However, proceed with caution.

Anal sex and teens: don't be an asshole!

Tell your teen: There is no rush to do this, no matter what you've seen in porn. Wait until you're really, really ready! When your teen does decide to embark upon this sexual journey, parents, I have some words of wisdom for you to share with them. The first is F (finger) before P (penis), and P always with C (condom). Compare your finger with a penis; an erect penis is way bigger. Let your partner get used to the anal play before you stick your penis in there. A finger can feel good, but a penis can hurt. There has to be some transition time between finger and penis.

Never go from A (anus) to V (vagina) without changing the C (condom). In other words, do not put the penis that was in the anus up the vagina without removing the condom, washing first, and putting on a new one. That is the fastest way to give your partner a yeast infection.

They will not thank you for that later. To repeat: do not go from A to V without changing the C.

Next: do not forget the lube. Lube is very important as this area is not naturally lubricated and anal sex can be very painful. Use K-Y Jelly or another condom-safe lube.

For safety reasons, remember that anal tissue is very delicate and therefore more prone to spread sexually transmitted infections! So again: use lube. If your teenager is a frequent rider on the A train and not monogamous, consider PrEP (pre-exposure prophylaxis, a drug that, when taken every day, can prevent the HIV infection that is becoming more and more common in the homosexual male community).

Now, on to consent. Parents, warn your teen that when they get consent ahead of time to go to a Mexican restaurant, it does not mean that their partner will want the whole enchilada. Pain during the process is common. When that time comes, pull out and reassess the situation. Although jokes are made about "surprise butt sex," reinforce that it is *never* appropriate to surprise anyone with *any* sexual activity–and, moreover, it is illegal as well as unethical. Remind your teen: just because you are playing with the asshole does not mean you need to be one.

6

Annihilating
the Risks

• • • •

Do you know how to use the tech your child uses?

• • • •

Technology holds much promise for improving communication, education, and leisure for us and our children. But technology can also pose new problems. According to Pew Research, "On average, 8- to 12-year-olds use just under five hours' worth of screen media per day and teens use an average of just under seven and a half hours' worth—not including time spent using screens for school or homework." To me, this is a shocking amount of time to spend glued to a device.

Parents should begin monitoring a child's access to technology, including cell phones, by the time the child is mobile. Kids learn quickly how to navigate computers, tablets, and phones, and while technology can be educational and fun, it is also easy for them to stumble upon things that are confusing or upsetting. Parental controls can play a critical role in ensuring your own privacy, as well as protecting your children from exposure to things that you would rather they did not see. Educate yourself on how parental controls operate. Private photos can be organized into password-protected folders, for example. Review ratings on video games and movies rather than taking your child's word for their appropriateness.

Children can often outfox their parents in terms of technology. I have heard numerous horror stories from friends and other parents about their children finding their technology and stealing passwords in order to read texts, or those old iCloud photos popping up at inopportune moments.

The takeaway here is, do not forget to completely wipe your old phones or tablets if you give them to your child, as they will probably know more than you do about how to find hidden content, even in their early years. Also, use technology to outsmart your kids. The newest apps such as Qustodio put smart programmers on your side so you can be sure you know what's going on with your kid's technology and that they cannot outsmart you as long as it is installed. They may be smarter than you, but the programmers in Silicon Valley are still smarter than them, so seek their help to keep your children safe.

Take inventory (on social media)
• • • •

Children have unprecedented access to the Internet, including social media, on their phones and tablets. If you do allow your child to have social media accounts, you should monitor them closely. Set time limits for the use of social media (no Instagram after 7 p.m., for example). As your child enters the teen years, monitoring their account and limiting their use will become increasingly more difficult. The trick then becomes figuring out a way to help ensure their safety and psychological well-being while also allowing them to develop and maintain a sphere of relatively private activity.

Be aware of shifting trends. Also be aware that social media platforms rapidly multiply, and what is popular amongst middle schoolers today may be completely passé tomorrow. As a friend's eighth grader told her, "Facebook is for old people." Some parents do not even know the wide variety of platforms that exist for sharing photos, videos, and comments.

Be aware of negative social comparison. Many social media platforms encourage social comparison, which can be unhealthy. Explain to children that people only post their best photos, the pictures of themselves in their best bathing suit from the best angle, so that they look the most desirable to others, and that sometimes they've taken dozens in order to get one perfect shot. This is not necessarily something that kids will realize. Some preteens and teens become obsessed with their online image, worrying about every photo or post. You should initiate discussion about what other teenagers are posting on their social media accounts, and about the values that are reflected in their activity. Some photos and videos are clearly bids for attention, so this can provide an opportunity to bring up the topics of body image, self-respect, and sexual desirability.

Do a monthly app inventory. Once a month, you should sit down with your child and go through all the applications that are downloaded on their phone. Ask them to show you the social media platforms that they use, or that other kids use, and ask them to show you the content on them. If you show interest in their world, rather than acting like a cop, they will be more likely to talk with you about social media. (But realize that they may also cleanse their phone if they know you are going to disapprove of something they have downloaded!)

I also recommend that you consider picking up their phone when they don't expect it and going through their texts and social media accounts. This makes sense for younger adolescents who are more at risk for rash decisions that have long-term consequences. I have found Snapchat to be especially problematic since the material erases quickly, and the only way to find out what is going on is to check the messages before they erase. I recommend that most parents forbid the use of this app. As far as the backlash from your teen? They should know that their phone is not private, as YOU pay for it, and *everything* is on the Internet. As they gain your trust, they might be able to expect more privacy from you and therefore less snooping. However, monitoring of their phone may keep them from saying or doing things they don't want you to see. Inappropriate material, whether posted by your child or one of their peers, can be an opportunity for discussion about your family's values, privacy, and the repercussions of sharing things online.

Keep an eye out for cyberbullying
· · · ·

Cyberbullying differs from regular bullying as it involves the use of the Internet to intimidate, stalk, or otherwise harass another child. I have seen it involve setting up a fake Instagram account (finsta) with the name of another child and then using the finsta to ruin the reputation of that child or bully another child. I have seen depressed teenagers being told to kill themselves online. One extreme case occurred in 2014 when Michelle Carter, aged 17, pressured her boyfriend to kill himself via a string of text messages; she was charged with involuntary manslaughter and convicted, and sentenced to 15 months in prison. There is a documentary on HBO called *I Love You, Now Die* on the subject. This is an extreme form of cyberbullying, but I have seen so many cases in my practice, ranging from gay bashing to mean-girl drama.

Cyberbullying, when directly or indirectly linked to suicide, has been referred to as "cyberbullicide." Dr. Sameer Hinduja and Dr. Justin Patchin reported results from a survey involving approximately 2,000 middle school children which indicated that victims of cyberbullying were almost twice as likely to attempt suicide as those who were not bullied. These results also indicated that cyberbullying offenders were 1.5 times as likely to report having attempted suicide compared with children who were not offenders or victims of cyberbullying. Although cyberbullying cannot be identified as a sole predictor of suicide in adolescents and young adults, it can increase risk of suicide by amplifying feelings of isolation, instability, and hopelessness for those with preexisting emotional, psychological, or environmental stressors.

I have seen suicidal thoughts, depression, and serious self-esteem issues that were directly linked to cyberbullying. Thankfully, I have also seen the schools in my community step up their watch of this, and begin monitoring the computer accounts of laptops and other devices given to students. There are frequent suspensions in the Hamptons schools for cyberbullying even on a child's personal computer/ phone. In one case the local police in the Hamptons got involved, and the student had to go through probation and hire a lawyer after sending a bullying email to a teacher. In this context, the educational and legal ramifications should be explained to teenagers.

Some tips to prevent cyberbullying? The most important is to make sure you are always monitoring your child's accounts and devices, and if you suspect your child is being bullied, try to reach out to the parent of the other child or to the school psychological support services to intervene, as things can quickly get very serious. If your child is the one who has sent the messages, a good old-fashioned apology note and a set amount of time spent grounded with suspension of devices is a great way to make sure they take it seriously. Also, how much trust you have in your child depends on their track record with their phone and social media use. If you catch them doing inappropriate things, I tell parents to take their child's phone once a month and just scroll through it and talk with the child about what is on it. Make sure you look at all of their social media accounts, and say that trust will be given when trust is earned, and that they can expect random checks of their devices. If they want privacy, get them a diary that they can put under their bed. It may result in a lot of screams and anger from the teen's end—but this is better than probation and legal issues.

A Patient's Story: John

JOHN, A 13-YEAR-OLD boy, posted a drawing of a teacher on his social media account, along with the text "Such a Fag." Many of his classmates were upset at the post and shared it with the teacher. The teacher, who was in fact homosexual, was horrified to see the post. John had interpreted his post as a relatively harmless one about the teacher, who was not well-liked among the teens. Up to that point, it had been common for boys to use slurs to put each other down. All the parents had tolerated the language, excusing it as "boys will be boys."

John was very remorseful, and he was suspended for several months. His action was reported to the local authorities, which resulted in legal bills and court dates. His parents expressed surprise and concern that the effects of his behavior had been so far-reaching. While I was happy that the school was addressing cyberbullying, I also felt sorry that John had to face so many consequences based on this one impulsive mistake. As parents, we must do a better job of curbing this kind of behavior before it gets out of hand and results in serious repercussions for the child and for other children.

Dispel distorted myths (caused by pornography)

• • • •

Before at least age 10, children cannot comprehend pornography as a fantasy. In the earliest years, a child may not even react; however, many children find pornographic images or videos to be upsetting or confusing if they are accidentally exposed to them. Sex may look like violence, for example, and it will not be easy to explain the difference. I prefer tight control over the possibility of accessing inappropriate content during these years. In early childhood and the tween years, pornography can have a negative impact on how children view sex. Parents should feel no shame about peering over their child's shoulder sometimes when they are on their devices, asking what they are watching. You should ask your child what they have been shown by friends, and whether other parents monitor them.

Younger children are more likely to feel confused and disturbed by pornography. Make sure that your young child understands that although you do not want them to look at these types of images, you will not get angry if they want to discuss something that they have accidentally seen. What I've actually found is that kids sometimes WANT to tell on other kids, so they don't have to look at things they don't like anymore. Parents should remember to change passwords, and to erase their web history after looking at pornography. An even easier solution is that most computers allow different logins and access to the hard drive for each user, and this can prevent these slipups from happening. (Perhaps you don't want your child looking at your bank statements or Word documents either.)

By middle school, exposure to pornography or sexualized media is inevitable, no matter how strictly you guard your child's access at home. Continue to reinforce the idea that they should approach you if they have questions or feel upset about something they have seen. Comparing pornography to watching a horror movie, you can remind them that it is difficult to get some images out of your head, and that your child may want to think carefully before watching something simply because other kids are.

Teenagers, the research shows, *do* end up watching pornography, regardless of what their parents believe and whether they actively seek it out or stumble across it by accident. Boys see porn more frequently by choice, but girls are also exposed. Many kids are involuntarily exposed to pornographic images by peers. One great study found that 93 percent of boys and 62 percent of girls viewed pornography during adolescence, suggesting that porn exposure is normative for teenagers. Only 12 percent of parents are aware of what their kids are watching. And they aren't just watching missionary sex scenes, according to a *New York Times Magazine* article; one soon-to-be-published study by Dr. Debby Herbenick and Dr. Bryant Paul, both fabulous sex researchers, found that 25 percent of girls and 36 percent of boys had seen "facials" (men ejaculating on women's faces), around 35 percent of both sexes had seen BDSM scenes, 20 percent of girls and 26 percent of boys had seen double penetration (one or more penises or objects in a woman's anus and/or vagina), and 31 percent of boys (and half that percentage of girls) had viewed "gang bangs," or group sex, and "rough oral sex" (a man aggressively thrusting his penis in and out of a mouth).

Not every porn viewer wants to act out what they have seen, although some older teens reported that they did (44 percent of males and 29 percent of females). A 2016 meta-analysis of pornography research reveals adolescent pornography consumption is significantly associated with stronger gender-stereotypical sexual beliefs, earlier sexual debut, increased casual sex behavior, and increased sexual aggression as both perpetrators and victims.

Even though most teens rated porn as unrealistic and even unappealing, this widespread exposure still indicates a need for more discussion about what pornography is and how to process it.

Parents do not need to watch porn with their teens to teach them to be more discerning viewers of all types of media.

A Patient's Story: Mark

ONE OF MY PATIENTS was a 12-year-old boy named Mark. He had a long history of obsessive-compulsive disorder—reflected in obsessing over germs, organizing his room, and washing his hands—which I treated successfully with cognitive behavioral therapy. As a preteen, he also developed the trademark symptom of obsessive-compulsive disorder, which is a need to confess. Every time he had a sexually inappropriate thought or masturbated, he felt the need to tell his mother. He also began to surf the Internet and access pornographic websites. He didn't even understand all of the sexual activities he was exposed to online, although he would watch them obsessively. When he told his mother what he had seen, it disturbed her as well. Through our ongoing clinical work, Mark began to realize that much of the content on the websites was detrimental to his well-being. He printed out pictures that were not disturbing to him but still sexually explicit— like a picture of an adult, naked woman—that he could use instead while masturbating.

A Patient's Story: **Gavin**

GAVIN, A 16-YEAR-OLD patient of mine, was attractive, athletic, and a good student. An all-American kid. He also watched plenty of pornography, beginning at age 12. His parents didn't set up any Internet filters and gave him his space. When he started having sex with his first girlfriend, Valerie, the impact of this habit began to manifest itself. He became very insecure about his penis size. His parents didn't walk around naked, and his lacrosse teammates did not get fully undressed in the locker room, so the penises he saw were the oversized penises in porn. He also learned from porn that women are very loud when they have sex, and that they like to be handled roughly. When Valerie asked him to use a softer touch, he was confused at first. Wasn't aggression what women liked? She showed him how to slow down and give her multiple orgasms, but Gavin was still dissatisfied. He longed to be with the big-breasted women he had conditioned himself to be aroused by in porn, not a teen girl with newly developing breasts. He just didn't feel as excited by Valerie. They stayed together for four months, and after their breakup he moved from girl to girl.

Gavin told me that he regretted watching so much porn because it made real sex less desirable than masturbation. We talked about what turned him on, and about how to evaluate porn scenes as performances. Real sex wouldn't be as loud or acrobatic. The angles wouldn't always make people look perfect.

Gavin still struggles with his identity and his sexuality. I have encouraged him to use pictures instead of pornography for arousal during masturbation and to focus on a girl's pleasure as the best way to connect sexually. He has had a girlfriend more recently, and has been putting her sexual needs above his own. He has learned to ask her questions about what she likes, and to delay his own orgasm for the sake of hers. These behaviors have proven to be a great self-esteem booster, as she has repeatedly told him "how good he is and how much she loves their sex." This has resulted in great improvement of his self-esteem, self-image, and ability to foster more healthy female attachments.

Gavin's story is *very* common with teens these days; his is not a rare case. The porn that kids are consuming now is hard-core. There is a controversial debate among psychologists and neuroscientists around sex addiction related to porn. The power of porn to deliver unending stimulation and a stream of novel sexual activities creates an incredible activation of our reward system. Because of this, there are theories that the excessive watching of porn is creating a supernormal stimuli. "Supernormal stimuli" is a term evolutionary biologists like Nobel Prize winner Nikolaas Tinbergen use to describe any stimulus that elicits a response more strongly than the stimulus for which the response evolved, even if the supernormal stimulus is artificial (such as Internet porn compared with real sex, or the sugar in candy compared with the sugar found in nature). This might help to explain why some people become addicted to junk food or porn at the expense of what's healthy for them.

To illustrate this, Tinbergen created artificial bird eggs that were larger and more colorful than actual bird eggs. Surprisingly, the mother birds chose to sit on the more vibrant artificial eggs and abandon their own naturally laid eggs. Similarly, Tinbergen created artificial butterflies with larger and more colorful wings, and male butterflies repeatedly tried to mate with these artificial butterflies in lieu of actual female butterflies. Supernormal stimuli activate our natural reward system, but potentially activate it at higher levels than the levels of activation our ancestors typically encountered as our brains evolved, making the brain liable to switch into an addictive mode. So some experts are saying that watching porn can make you want novel stimulation and can make regular sex less rewarding.

The free porn that children are able to watch (from Pornhub, for example) can be extremely violent: "88.2% contained physical aggression, principally spanking, gagging, and slapping, while 48.7% of scenes contained verbal aggression, primarily name-calling. Perpetrators of aggression were usually male, whereas targets of aggression were overwhelmingly female. Targets most often showed pleasure or responded neutrally to the aggression." In her book *Pornland*, Dr. Gail Dines, a professor of sociology and expert on this subject, writes: "The messages that porn disseminates about women can be boiled down to a few essential characteristics: they are always ready for sex and are enthusiastic to do whatever men want, irrespective of how painful, humiliating, or harmful the act is. The word 'no' is glaringly absent from porn women's vocabulary." Dr. Dines says in an interview on NPR's *On Point* that you can liken the porn industry to a predatory capitalist industry—insidiously trying to get teenagers hooked early on so that they become lifelong users. She feels it is like handing out free cigarettes to middle schoolers. If teens have access to free hard-core porn from very early ages, the more long-term effects there may be.

The free porn that most kids have access to is much more graphic and violent than the porn you have to pay for. And it is also less likely to be made ethically, with fair trade practices (fair wages, basic health coverage, and STI testing). There are some resources out there to help you find fair trade porn. Literotica is pornography you read—like the stories we used to secretly devour in our parent's copy of *Playboy*. It can stimulate the imagination without the sometimes disturbing images. Other websites like EroticFilms, PinkLabel, and Four Chambers are places to find more ethically made pornography. But chances are that if you have not paid for the pornography, then it most likely is not ethically made. How you want to handle this issue as a parent is a personal choice. Would you allow your late teen to buy porn, or would you forbid it? For early teens the answer is easier, but with later teens it can get more tricky, as they may be using it anyway, no matter what you say.

Parental involvement is critical in how children receive and perceive porn. My advice is that we should do our best to keep children under the age of 14 away from pornography by monitoring their technology. After that age, they need to be given the freedom to make their own choices, as they will find a way to get what they want in any case. There are some great resources for parents about pornography on the website Culture Reframed (culturereframed.org). There are also books, such as *Good Pictures Bad Pictures: Porn-Proofing Today's Young Kids* by Kristen A. Jenson and Debbie Fox, that are meant for tweens and teens and may help set the stage for the discussion.

The best way you can combat the likelihood of your teen getting addicted to or suffering the negative consequences of watching pornography is by talking about it, and getting ahead of it with some major myth busters!

Top 5 things to tell your teenager about pornography

1   **Most pornography is acting.** Maybe some healthy adults have sex in these ways, but most probably do not. The camera angles, lighting, and flow of sexual activity are part of an overall production process. Sometimes, porn falsely portrays activities that could be as painful as they are pleasurable. Other times, porn portrays activities that may be pleasurable in ways that look uncomfortable or painful. Orgasms and ejaculations can be faked. They might also sometimes be real, in the same way that an actress's tears are "real" during an emotional scene in a regular film.

2   **Most people's bodies do not look like the bodies of porn actors and actresses.** Porn performers are chosen because of certain physical attributes (large penises, oversized breasts) that sell videos. Many times, actors and actresses have altered their bodies through cosmetic surgical procedures.

3 **If pornography is upsetting you, don't continue watching it.**
Sometimes teens may group together and watch lascivious scenes
through peer pressure, but your child can choose to leave or stop
watching. It is impossible to "unsee" something you've seen, and
it might be difficult to get a pornographic scene out of your mind
when you begin to have real sex. You could see some beautiful,
erotic things, but you might also see some awful things. Think
before you click. The effect can be compared to that of a horror
film that gave you nightmares: it was not worth it in the end, so
just walk out of the room, turn your back, and say, "I don't want
to watch this," or turn off the screen.

4 **Pornography often displays less common, or "fringe," sex acts.**
Most people do not, or at least do not *often*, engage in this kind
of sex, and certainly not until they are older and more mature
and know their boundaries. Most teenagers are not ready for such
things. Tell your child to focus on intimacy and connection in their
sexual encounters, as there will be plenty of time for the other
stuff later if they so choose.

5 **Consent! Porn performers are asked to give consent before
shooting a scene, even if they do not give consent onscreen.**
Remember that they are acting; just like WWE wrestlers, they may
have rehearsed their moves. Don't assume, because a porn actor
reaches out and slaps an actress during sex, that this is acceptable
in real life. Never assume that slapping, pinching, or other "rough
sex" activities are automatically consented to as part of intercourse. Never assume that anal sex is consented to just because
you are having vaginal sex. And remember that porn performers
are professionals–you might not see them using lubricant or discussing safety measures, but most of the time these things *are*
happening offscreen.

Lead with the legalities (on sexting)

• • • •

Sexting, or sending nude or seminude photos through text messages or mobile applications, is increasingly common among teens. (One-quarter of youth are sexting.) Parents, don't have ostrich syndrome when it comes to sexting. Studies show that teens who sext are more likely to be sexually active and have multiple sex partners, tend not to use contraception, are more likely to have delinquent behavior and internalizing problems, and have higher rates of substance use. The younger they start sexting, the higher these risks are.

Why do preteens become involved in sexting? Motivations range: desiring attention, rebelling, pleasing a boyfriend or girlfriend, wanting to feel more grown-up, thinking it is "funny," wanting revenge, curiosity, and so on. Some teens have admitted to being pressured or even bullied to take or share photos. Yet experts agree that not only do kids fail to grasp the permanence of digital imagery, they also fail to understand the legal implications.

Parents should warn their kids as soon as they begin using such technology about the dangers of sending images; after all, it isn't just nude photos that can create backlash once they are made public—even years after the fact. Sexting has implications for personal privacy but also becomes a consent violation if photos are forwarded to unintended recipients. As of 2016, 20 states had laws regulating sexting. In some states, if the photos are of underage individuals, the person who sent them then becomes susceptible to charges of child pornography. After an investigation in Virginia that implicated more than 100 teenagers and more than 1,000 photos of nude or seminude teens on cell phones and social media sites, local authorities argued that "age-appropriate" training was necessary at the middle school level, not just in high schools.

Teens these days are getting a lot of their information online; from porn to sexting, they are living in a virtual world. This creates real gaps when it comes to forming actual relationships, to the detriment of your child. Your child should be encouraged to be intimate in real time. This is the better way to encourage them to have healthy intimate relationships in the future. This means you must be comfortable with having conversations about sex, and set guidelines around where they are allowed to have it–the safest place being in your home. This will allow them to express their sexuality in a healthier, safer way than by sending online images (see "How should you handle your teenager having sex in the home?," page 140). Once you establish these ground rules, you will have credibility when you ask them to be careful about sexting, because if you tell them they cannot date–or have sex–they will go behind your back and live in a virtual world. If, on the other hand, you don't feel they are ready or mature enough for real sex, then there must be a real discussion about it.

Don't have ostrich syndrome and thereby force them to seek out intimacy in a virtual world. Better to have a real conversation, assess their safety, provide contraception, and ask that they be careful with what they do online. Of course, you should also monitor their social media and all Internet accounts until you are really confident they can be responsible, as the consequences can be disastrous.

5 tips on sexting for teens

1 Do flirt! On texts, this can be a great way to connect. Combine flattery and gentle teasing as a great way to flirt in order to establish a new connection. (See flirting training section on page 122.)

2 Do send alluring but not naked pictures—nothing that reveals the nipples or genitals.

3 If you want to get really sexy, then use a phone call/FaceTime. It can be recorded, but it is less likely to be kept and forwarded.

4 Snapchat videos do not really disappear, I promise, so educate your child that this is not a safe way to communicate.

5 Sexy time is best done in person. This is the ideal way to really be intimate. Parents, let your child know they can come to you and you can help them create a safe space to get intimate rather than doing it online.

Instill "No friend left behind" (with drugs and partying)
• • • •

As with sex, strict prohibitions do not always work to prevent substance use. Parents should explain the dangers of alcohol and drug use accurately and realistically, rather than using sensationalized and easily disproved claims such as, "You'll die if you do a line of cocaine" or "One puff and you're addicted for life." At the same time, explain the legal ramifications of substance use, which can range from misdemeanors to expulsion from school to loss of driving privileges. Remember that if your teenager invites friends over to drink or use substances without your knowledge, you could be liable if something goes wrong.

Your teen should understand that intoxication affects decision-making and can lead to incapacitation. Teens might want to set up a buddy system so that they do not abandon friends who are drunk or high. Parents can insist on a "no friend left behind" policy–and help their teens carry it out through open communication. Teen girls should be advised to never leave a friend alone with a person they have just met–and never to put themselves in such a situation. Sticking together can help avoid many dangerous situations. If they feel a romantic interest after meeting someone, your child should exchange information first, and then they can make plans to see each other again at another time.

I've heard this story too many times, both in my practice and while working in medical environments: girl drinks heavily, meets boy, separates from her friends, and ends up in a coercive situation.

A Patient's Story: Sara

AT 16, ONE OF my patients named Sara accompanied her girlfriends to a high school party. She met a boy who was in his first year of college. Everyone did shots, including Sara. When the boy asked her to go to another party, she said yes immediately. Her friends were reluctant to let her go, but she insisted. They could see that Sara was really into him, and he was older, handsome, attending a good college—everything they too would want in a boyfriend. But instead of taking her to another party, he took her back to his house. By that time, Sara was quite drunk. He coerced her into sex. Although he didn't use force, he didn't need to. Sara knew she couldn't get home easily. She didn't even know where she was. So she closed her eyes and hoped that it would end quickly. It did, and then he drove her home.

In the morning, she woke up physically sore and emotionally distraught. She wondered if she should tell someone, but decided to keep it to herself—until she told me. I explained that although it wasn't her fault, it also would not have happened if she had not been intoxicated, or if she had not split off from her friends. Sara committed to me—but most importantly to herself—to always stay with her friends, and to remind herself that if the guy was worth it, he would take her on a real date at another time. She realized that this kind of spontaneous, intoxicated sex made her feel worse about herself rather than empowered or desirable. She feels more in control of her body now, and more confident in her interactions.

Yes, in a perfect world, date rape or unwanted sex would not be consequences of getting too drunk—for women or men. But we do not yet live in that perfect world, and until then we need to be realistic.

Parents must stress that consent cannot be given by someone who is intoxicated, and that continuing with sexual activity in this context not only is bad manners but can result in very serious consequences for all involved. The idea that men get women drunk to entice them to take off their clothes is sadly a reality in our society, and it is tied to the idea of the "walk of shame"—the regret and disgust that follows decisions made in such a sex-negative context. Remind your teen that you will help them out of a bind if they do something stupid, or if they witness their peers making mistakes. If they know you have their back, they are more likely to have the strength to do the right thing.

Make sure your teenager realizes that if someone is so drunk or high that they are falling down, passing out, or nonresponsive, not seeking help can be fatal and even criminal. Tragic stories abound about situations that might easily have been prevented. Jordan Johnson, an 18-year-old from East Hampton, made the news not for his athletic accomplishments but because he overdosed at a "party home." When he arrived at the hospital, unconscious, in kidney failure, and breathing with the help of a ventilator, he was put into a medically induced coma. Johnson had been "passed out" on the ground for more than 12 hours before a call to 911 was placed the following morning; a Snapchat video posted at 8 p.m. showed him lying unconscious while other teens shouted into his ear with a megaphone to rouse him. It is hard to imagine the callousness of a teenager who chooses to laugh and Snapchat a video rather than seek medical attention for a friend—or even a stranger. But for adolescents, the combination of peer pressure, intoxication, fear, and the desire to be popular—even to generate "likes" on social media—can be powerful.

A Patient's Story: **Ryan**

RYAN WAS A 17-YEAR-OLD boy who came into my office because he was overwhelmed with anxiety, sadness, and feelings of social inadequacy. He felt ugly, and described himself as a "loser" because his best friend got more attention from, and was even able to "score" more easily with, girls at school. To give himself "liquid courage," Ryan began drinking before every social event. Drunkenness allowed him to forget about his shame and insecurities ("no girl will find me attractive"), but when he was successful at finding a girl to have sex with, he barely remembered the experience. Unfortunately, the drinking progressed to an addiction that was harder to treat than his original complaints. He began to have blackouts, and would drive after drinking.

No matter how many sexual experiences Ryan had, his self-esteem remained low. Having sex did not rid him of feelings of inferiority or inadequacy. When I suggested that he focus on the pleasurable aspects of the sexual experience rather than the competition, he became agitated. "Dr. L, I have to prove to my friends that I'm not ugly and not a loser."

Ryan's parents were divorced, and disagreed vehemently about how to handle his anxiety (among many other things). His father was harsh, concerned about his son's drinking, but not serving as an example for Ryan in his own relationships with women, which tended to be frequent and short-lived. Ryan's mother was overly permissive, often ignoring his "bad boy" behavior. With neither parent confronting him about how he treated women sexually, he not only lacked guidance in navigating relationships but had begun to dehumanize women—and himself.

Through our sessions, Ryan eventually came to understand that competing with his friends was making him feel worse. Through his continual comparisons of himself with others, he kept creating "shoulds": he should be better-looking, he should get more girls, he should exercise more, he should go further when he hooked up. Through cognitive behavioral therapy, we worked on changing his thought patterns and defeating core negative beliefs linking dating rejection directly to his sense of self-worth. He developed a new approach: "you need to kiss a lot of frogs before you find your princess." Instead of gossiping with his friends about who they hooked up with, he focused on making better friendships. When he did find a sexual partner, he focused on giving her pleasure. Becoming an excellent lover gave him satisfaction and raised his self-esteem.

7

Teaching Radical Inclusion for Gender, Sexual, & Family Identities and Expressions

● ● ● ●

Gender and sexual identity and expression

. . . .

Parents, you need to teach your children from a young age about gender and sexual orientation, and do so in a developmentally appropriate way. It will be important to stress that gender identity is fluid and expressed in many ways (girls can wear pants and boys can wear dresses even in the mainstream, i.e., kilts). It will also be important to explain that you can be outside the box in terms of your gender expression but still identify as the sex you were born with, such as men who like to sport long hair or wear feminine clothing but still identify as men, or women who have very short hair and look more masculine but still identify as women. This can be explained easily, and kids get it. The more fluid and accepting you are as a parent, the easier it will be for your child to feel comfortable taking on both masculine and feminine traits. We'll look at the reasons for acceptance in the section "Allow your child to 'try on' a gender."

You can start with the basic definitions below, which can be explained to children starting at age seven.

Defining the terms

Biological sex: The sex you were assigned at birth based on your physical genitalia and your chromosomal makeup. Females have two X chromosomes and males have an X and a Y chromosome. In rare cases, an individual will be categorized as "intersex," or having chromosomal or physical abnormalities of varying degrees.

Cisgender: Your gender identity matches the sex you were assigned by parents/doctors at birth.

Gender: The cultural and social expectations and norms around being male and female.

Gender expression: How people express characteristics of their gender on their body (clothing, hairstyle, etc.) and through their actions or movements. Gender expression is fluid and can change over time and over a person's life.

Gender identity: Someone's personal sense of themselves as a man or woman (or both, or neither). Gender identity begins forming at around age three, and is usually fairly stable over the life course. Most people are "cisgender," which means their gender identity matches the sex they were assigned at birth. Some people, however, identify as transgender, meaning that their gender identity does not match the sex they were assigned at birth. Other people do not like to be labeled at all, and may use terms such as "gender non-binary" or "gender-queer" to describe themselves. Neutral pronouns, such as "they/ze/sie" (rather than "he" or "she"), may be preferred by people who do not identify as cisgender.

Sexual orientation: Your pattern of attraction to partners, whether to individuals of the same sex (homosexual), the opposite sex (heterosexual), or both sexes (bisexual). Some people use the term "asexual," meaning that they do not experience sexual attraction to anyone; others use the term "pansexual," which means they are attracted to people with a variety of gender expressions.

Transgender: Your gender identity does not match the sex you were assigned by parents/doctors at birth.

Explaining sexual and gender diversity for all ages

Giving youth some vocabulary to describe themselves and the people they meet will help them understand more about themselves, just as giving children knowledge of the names of their body parts will help them protect themselves from sexual assault.

It will also help every child, regardless of their identity, understand their peers and the adults they may encounter who are transgender, and be accepting of that community. Even young children often show curiosity about families that are different from their own, and increasing family diversity means that they may encounter nontraditional family types by preschool if they are not already living in one.

This is a good time to start explaining the differences between gender expression and sexual identity. Terms like "tomboy" reflect differences in gender expression, while terms like "transgender" represent differences in gender identity–but both refer to people who do not fit stereotypical gender expectations.

In my practice, I've found that being open with children about the diversity of people they encounter will help them be more accepting and loving. Openness will also prevent a self-esteem crisis if they realize that *they* fall outside the box. Language and knowledge can empower them to describe their desires and experiences. I have not found that these discussions push kids towards alternative lifestyles, but rather free them from anguish and isolation.

If the issue has not arisen earlier, parents should make sure that children understand that gender and sexual diversity exists, and that kids learn how to handle interactions with someone who is different from the people they have previously encountered.

Just as kids should be told not to use words like "fag" or "pussy" to humiliate other kids, let them know that even using words like "gay" or "queer" as negative adjectives is hugely problematic. These words can hurt the person they are used against, and offend people who identify as LGBTQ+ (or know people who do).

If your child claims to have a non-heterosexual or nonnormative gender identity, or if you suspect that will be the case in the future, it is important to familiarize yourself with some of the issues that can arise due to misunderstanding and stigma, from bullying to depression.

Great relationships start with great role models

• • • •

The early years are often marked by an intense interest in the composition of one's own family, gender roles, and relationships. Your child is always learning through observation, and this includes observations about the division of labor in your household, how disagreements are handled, who makes decisions, and so on. Be mindful of the unconscious lessons that your child is absorbing from your everyday life.

The case for an opposite-sex role model

Opposite-sex role models are important during infancy and the toddler years. At a time when the naturalness of gender roles, and even biological sex, is being challenged from many angles, it might seem dated to suggest that spending time with an individual of the opposite sex is important to a child's development. Yet the reality of the world is still that most people identify as either masculine or feminine, and regardless of a child's own identity, or the identity of their parents, they will encounter people who fall into both categories, so it is important for them to interact with someone from the opposite end of the gender/sexuality spectrum.

I believe that opposite-sex role models can help children navigate the world in other ways than just sexually, and that children who lack them can grow up at a disadvantage. Sigmund Freud believed that children fall in love with the opposite-sex parent but then transfer that relationship onto opposite-sex partners later in life after they realize that a parent is an unacceptable sex partner. Although I believe his theories of the Oedipal and Electra complexes go too far by suggesting that children want to harm the same-sex parent, I do believe that there is a process of identification that occurs, and that this impacts a child's ability to form healthy, trusting relationships later in their life.

Opposite-sex role models should not simply be understood as providing examples of "male" or "female" behavior, but also as a way to combat cultural stereotypes. Adult men can model respect and empathy for young girls, showing that these are qualities for both men and women to display. If a young girl is exposed to a loving male figure, she will develop expectations for how men can treat women. This is a win-win, because even if the child doesn't pick members of the opposite sex as intimate partners, they are still going to have to work and interact with the opposite sex in their day-to-day life, and should have high standards in ALL environments for how they are treated by this opposite sex.

Plenty of children, of course, grow up without any male role models, though far fewer without any female role models, and end up well-adjusted. Some children grow up with negative male or female role models, such as parents who are inattentive or abusive or who have severe psychological issues. My argument is not that development is impossible without opposite-sex role models, just that there is a place for such a contrast in a child's life.

What to do if you suspect your child is outside the box

• • • •

The statistics

Sexual minority youth are those who identify as gay, lesbian, bisexual, queer, transgender—anything other than heterosexual. In a recent study by the CDC, 88 percent of high school students identified as heterosexual, 2 percent identified as gay or lesbian, 6 percent identified as bisexual, and 3.2 percent were not sure of their sexual identity. Identifying as other than heterosexual was not necessarily related to having had same-sex (or opposite-sex) contact: in the same study, 48 percent of students had had sexual contact with only the opposite sex, 1.7 percent had had sexual contact with only the same sex, 4.6 percent had had sexual contact with both sexes, and 45.7 percent had had no sexual contact.

Many sexual minority youth cope adequately with the pressures of childhood and adolescence, but as a whole they are vulnerable to stigma, discrimination, bullying, familial and social rejection, and increased risks of violence. Forced sexual intercourse was higher among gay, lesbian, and bisexual students (17.8 percent) and not-sure students (12.6 percent) than heterosexual students (5.4 percent). Young gay and bisexual males are at increased risk for HIV and other STIs. It is very important to educate your teen about anal sex rather than avoiding the topic, as this type of sex does present a very particular set of health risks. Sexual minority youth are also at increased risk for depression and even suicide.

Allow your child to "try on" a gender

For parents who suspect that their young child may be questioning their gender identity or sexual orientation, my advice is to be prepared to "bend at the knees." My experience is that children can bounce back and forth during childhood and adolescence. I have seen "tomboy" girls who hate wearing dresses and choose only to play with boys grow up to become cisgender (their biological sex matches their gender expression). I have also seen the opposite-gender expression persist into adolescence, and with that a desire to change their biological sex (transgender). Although long-term research on childhood gender dysphoria (feeling sadness or internal turmoil about their gender) is limited and politically controversial, in practice there are more options every year for kids who are questioning their sexual orientation and gender identity.

Steering your child towards solutions that are not permanent in order to try them out can be a useful first approach. When there is a great deal of emphasis placed on gender differences in the home, children suffer more when their gender expression does not match their biological sex. Keeping gender-neutral toys in the home, allowing children to choose their clothing without regard to gender, and allowing both boys and girls to express a variety of masculine and feminine traits is a healthier approach overall. Allow your child to wear their hair the way they feel most comfortable with or play with the toys they are drawn to. Having this freedom can actually prevent gender dysphoria. Children who are not allowed to explore beyond narrow, stereotypical gendered choices may eventually develop discomfort with their gender identity, resulting in depression and suicidal tendencies.

Some well-meaning parents and therapists support early transitioning with prevention of puberty and hormones, although I tend to think that many of these young children or adolescents need more time. Transitioning too quickly—and then changing one's mind—can be just as emotionally and physically challenging as being pushed to accept a gender that feels oppressive. In some cases, however, it is clear from the beginning that transitioning early will be the best strategy. Such decisions must be made on a case-by-case basis, with great thought put into risks and benefits of all options.

When parents resist a child's desire to explore gender options, I have noticed that it becomes difficult to disentangle whether a child is truly unhappy with their biology or whether they are rebelling against restrictions on their freedom of expression. Cultural trends such as the mainstreaming of the "emo" subculture in the early 2000s also affect gender expression in that generation. Emo developed out of 1980s hard-core punk, and is characterized by emotional and confessional lyrics. People who participated in emo subculture also developed particular androgynous fashion styles—skinny jeans, dark hair with bangs, black fingernails on boys and girls—and became associated with sensitivity, introversion, and even depression. Some parents interpret the adoption of such subcultural styles as gender confusion, although their child may simply be experimenting with different forms of self-expression rather than experiencing gender dysphoria.

But if you suspect—or know—that your child does not identify as heterosexual or cisgender, there are a number of steps that you can take to mitigate the risks of gender dysphoria. Many organizations exist that can help parents and children/adolescents navigate this landscape. Although I cannot delve too deeply into this topic here, parents who are faced with an actual case of gender dysphoria or a child's desire to transition should make certain to locate a professional psychiatrist with experience with such cases. There are also wonderful facilities to help educate you and your family about the various stages of transitioning to another gender and about the risks and benefits of each procedure. One such place is the Mount Sinai Center for Transgender Medicine and Surgery. Whether your child will "grow out" of nonconforming gender desires or will eventually want to transition, you will want experienced guidance along the way.

A Patient's Story: Chrissy

ONE OF MY PATIENTS, Chrissy, decided at the age of three that she felt more like a boy than a girl. Her parents, who are forward-thinking, wanted to get my advice on how to handle this in a sensitive way. At age five, she expressed the desire for the "peepee fairy" to bring her a penis. She demanded boys' clothes and that her hair be cut short—and her parents acquiesced. She preferred to have boys as friends and play sports like basketball.

Yet her gender identity was complex. When I asked her at age nine if she would prefer to use boys' or girls' bathrooms, she thought for a moment and then decided that she preferred girls' bathrooms. I asked about whether she wanted to use a male name, and again she stated that she preferred her own name. She told me that she understood she was a girl, and didn't want to change that even though she preferred to play with boys and dress like a boy.

I made sure that Chrissy understood that she could tell me if she was feeling at odds with her body and gender development, but she did not seem particularly stressed about either. To me, she seemed like a young girl interested in enjoying certain activities, thinking more about how she could best participate in the rough-and-tumble play that she loved than about how she was presenting herself to the world.

Chrissy was lucky to have parents who supported her decisions and did not make a big deal about them. In public, they often referred to Chrissy and her sister as "kids" or "kiddo" to avoid gendered language. Her school was also supportive. At one point, Chrissy read the book *Sex Is a Funny Word*, which briefly addresses the topic of transgender identities. She was not upset by the book, and only slightly interested. She is similarly not bothered when people mistake her for a boy, usually answering, "Yeah, I look like a boy, but I'm a girl."

Currently, Chrissy and her parents are still maintaining a "wait and see" attitude towards her gender identity. I believe that she will probably consider transitioning later on, though I want to make sure that she completely understands the ramifications of doing so if she takes that route. On the other hand, she may continue to identify as a woman who just happens to have a masculine appearance. Either way, the fact that her parents have maintained an attitude of acceptance means that Chrissy is a happy child with lots of friends of both genders, a variety of interests, and a healthy relationship with her body.

When your family is outside the box

• • • •

Nontraditional parents must work to create loving and respectful environments, just as other parents must, by fostering healthy, honest communication and maintaining clear boundaries. Nontraditional parents also find themselves confronted with unique challenges, whether practical, legal, social, or spiritual. How should parents explain their familial arrangements to their children at different ages, for example, especially given that the structure of a family inevitably raises the specter of sexuality?

Facing discrimination

Even something as simple as an elementary school playdate, or a neighborhood Mother's Day brunch, potentially becomes complicated for parents who do not fit the social majority, given that alternative family arrangements may be subjected to social scrutiny, if not outright stigma or legal difficulties. For example, the current immigration laws discriminate against same-sex couples who have babies using surrogates or sperm donors outside the US, sometimes denying the baby US citizenship. Even if the parents are married and live in the US, if the donor is not American, citizenship can be denied. Nontraditional parents, whether they wish to or not, challenge social norms and beliefs that are widespread and often institutionalized. This includes marriage, other legal systems (identification, inheritance, employment benefits, etc.), the medical system, the educational system, and so on.

In the courts and in the media, concerns about children growing up in families with single, divorced, or same-sex parents have repeatedly been raised. Will the children be poorly psychologically adjusted? Will they grow up heterosexual or gay? Will the social stigma of having single, divorced, or sexual minority parents lead to behavioral or emotional problems, either as children or adults? And given that adopted children face certain challenges, and that same-sex couples are about five times more likely to be raising adopted children, would this compound their vulnerability? How can parents help children explain their family to others—relatives, neighbors, teachers, or peers—in ways that are developmentally appropriate, culturally sensitive, respectful of personal privacy, and yet still factually accurate?

These stigmas are baseless!

Family structure itself does not inherently affect a child's development or future success. Just as we no longer think that the child of divorced parents is always going to develop social or psychological problems, we have learned to see the complexities involved with other family arrangements as well.

Overall, comparisons of gay, lesbian, and heterosexual parents have found few differences in psychological adjustment and mental health of the parents, parenting stress, and parental competence. For example, same-sex couples are actually more likely to share child care, housework, and paid employment than different-sex couples. Yet, just as single parents face some unique environmental, social, and financial challenges, same-sex parents experience parental issues if they live in less supportive legal contexts or receive less social support due to their sexual orientation; and even in contexts where they are supported, these parents may still encounter more child behavior problems. So it is not the parental arrangement that causes any familial issue; it is actually the lack of systemic and community support that causes strain.

Special issues for adoptive parents

Adoptive children represent about 1 percent of all children living in the US. Many books have been written on parenting adopted children. Because there are so many available resources (see the Notes section), I do not address every issue here but rather focus on special issues related to parenting and sexuality. There are studies supporting the notion that children adopted by same-sex parents are as well-adjusted as adopted children of heteronormative parents. No matter the sex of the parents, however, there are some issues that might come up earlier or more profoundly with adopted children, as discussed below.

Sex education might come up earlier with adoptive children, especially if they are aware that they are adopted or if they are of a different ethnicity from their parents. Adoptive parents may feel nervous answering questions about reproduction, and might not want to answer complicated questions about why some parents adopt rather than having their own biological children. Adoptive parents may also have little information about their child's birth story, which may have been a result of rape, teenage pregnancy, or an unknown father. If the child was adopted at some point after infancy, there may have been trauma (known or unknown) that the adoptive parents do not want to revisit.

A Patient's Story: **Michael**

MICHAEL IS A YOUNG boy in my practice who showed very poor boundaries after his adoption at age nine. He had a reactive attachment disorder, and was often very inappropriate with the male and female role models in his life, such as teachers, uncles, and his older step-siblings. Several times, Michael was caught creating fake social media aliases and communicating with older women on Facebook. He was also caught surfing the Internet for inappropriate sexual images and pornography, both at home and at school.

His pre-adoption history was very unclear, but I believed that he had possibly been sexually abused. He did not understand boundaries between himself and the adults around him, something that we see in children who have been sexually abused. Children who have been sexually abused also tend to be more sexually explicit and promiscuous. I suggested that, in addition to frequent monitoring of his computer and phone time, his adoptive mother should talk with him about sex, reproduction, and what he had seen online. He did not have enough information to satisfy his curiosity about sex and to put it in the right perspective, so he was finding less appropriate ways to get information. Telling him the correct information about sex, as well as letting him know that his job was just to be a kid right now and that sex was for later, was very reassuring for him, and he did not subsequently seek out information about sex in inappropriate ways.

Michael's story is extreme. However, it illustrates the point that adoptive parents may need to think well ahead of time about how to handle questions from their child about the adoption. Parents may also need to consider how to address and explain traumatic events that occurred before the adoption, ideally with the guidance of a professional clinician.

I believe in taking a no-nonsense approach to the issue of adoption from the start, explaining, from the time that a child can understand, that the sperm and the egg can come from a different set of parents. Distinguishing between birth parents and parents in biological terms allows the child to ask questions but also develop an understanding of how and why an individual might have more than one set of parents. Even if you do not know the reasons that your child was put up for adoption, you can discuss some of the reasons that birth (or biological) parents might not be ready to raise a child: their ages, a lack of resources, and so on.

Explaining nontraditional family arrangements for all ages

You may find that all of this "explaining" is more of an issue for parents, as kids can be very accepting! But taking into account all the common concerns outlined at the beginning of this chapter, it's important to consider how your children can explain their family to outsiders and peers, and to talk to them about it, to address the issue of "explaining," however arbitrary it may be to you. Take the time to help your children understand what types of things you feel they can share about their family situation and what should remain private.

Explaining same-sex parenting often requires explaining the different ways that reproduction can happen (sex or technology) or that families can form through adoption or remarriage after divorce, for example. You can explain that both male and female same-sex couples may use artificial insemination or in vitro fertilization to conceive, adopt, or have children from previous heterosexual unions. You could also explain that women can bear their own children if they so choose, while men still need to hire a surrogate if they choose to use reproductive technologies.

A Patient's Story: Gabbi

GABBI AND MOLLY had an unusual conception story. They both had eggs removed, and then fertilized them with sperm that was selected from a sperm bank. From 12 fertilized eggs, they picked the strongest one without knowing who the genetic mother was. Gabbi carried the fetus to term and their son, Harry, was born healthy. Since they live in California and are legally married, Molly did not need to adopt Harry but could be listed on the birth certificate.

Gabbi sometimes gets annoyed when people continually ask who the mother of the baby is. "They immediately want to know whose egg it was. They're like, well, 'It's Molly, he looks like Molly.' But maybe he looks like the sperm donor? We don't know. It's a very personal question, I think, but people from all walks of life and cultures ask. I say we are both mothers, end of story."

In a cultural setting where a parent-child relationship is assumed to be biological, different types of kinship ties can be confusing to people. But although people may ask some insensitive questions, you should not always assume malicious intent. Individuals from older generations may not have had much exposure to adoptive, same-sex, or otherwise nonnormative families. It is certainly not your job to explain the "new normal" to them, but taking the time to do so occasionally can also change the world, one person at a time. Nontraditional parents might develop a scripted response for these situations that is easy to give and feels genuine without allowing for outside intrusions.

Communities vary in terms of how open-minded residents are about sexuality. In some cities, same-sex parents would not even be notable at the playground or a school event with their child. In a small rural town, however, such a family could face varying degrees of hostility and prejudice. Nontraditional families will occasionally encounter resistance in less conservative communities as well. Even with regard to sex education, parents may find themselves at odds with others.

A Human Story: Omar

I INTERVIEWED OMAR, who is 18 years old and in a nontraditional family.

"My parents were outside the box, and it could be hard at times. If you live in San Francisco, where there is an extremely liberal population, it would be better to know from the beginning that your parents were poly[amorous]. So many people are accepting of that lifestyle there. But for my siblings and me, we at one point moved from the city to a Waspy suburban community, where it was much harder to be out of the norm, especially since we were not bursting with self-confidence—none of us were at the time.

"We already felt different enough in a metropolitan environment, we didn't need to feel like we were freaks in an even more conservative environment. Some people will embrace that, but it depends on the kid. Now, people accept me for being a divergent character, but in younger teen years, people are so insecure and I only wanted to tell people close to me like my best friends [about my family]. You need to have an understanding of your kid and their social scene, and you can judge when your kid has enough self-confidence to understand things, and reinforce the idea of love in all respects.

"In my really Waspy environment, I was able to understand what being different is like even though I'm, like, completely straight myself. I could understand what being gay and lesbian is all about. My parents also enforced that the idea of love can happen in all forms and you just need to let it happen. Their lifestyle taught me to be a divergent character, which I identify with, and to be more accepting of others."

There are places where nontraditional families can find support. But for the more vanilla parents out there, it can be easy to make assumptions about people's family life, for example saying something like, "Is your husband tall?" (I get this all the time as I am so tall that people want to make sure I am not with a shorter guy). A remark such as "Your mother and father should be proud of you" is making many assumptions: that the person has a mother and a father (not a same-sex couple or single-parent arrangement). It would be better to use gender-neutral language: "your *parents* should be proud" or "*they* must be good people." Teach your children to avoid offending or putting people in an awkward position by not making assumptions and not using gendered language. We should do our best to put other people at ease so they feel at liberty to share about their family life rather than becoming shut down or embarrassed about their situation.

Lastly, don't be afraid to apologize if you got it wrong or made the wrong assumption. Asking for clarification, and a little bit of apologetic naïveté, can go a long way.

8

A Parent's Ongoing Sexual Story

How your sexual story affects your child

• • • •

Now that we've talked about your kids and their sexuality, let's talk about yours and what it's okay to disclose when talking about sex with your child! We'll also talk about family disclosures to the world, dealing with different parenting arrangements, conflicts, divorce issues such as moving between households, and dealing with dating and the introduction of new partners. Let's look at real-world examples, and common issues that we all know people are experiencing across the board but we may not be hearing about very often.

Parent disclosures to children

• • • •

Psychiatrists are required to think carefully about the issue of disclosure and privacy. If I share something about my personal life with a patient, that information should be beneficial to the patient. But oversharing, or sharing without a specific purpose, could harm our therapeutic relationship. Oversharing can also potentially lead to a situation where the patient takes on the role of therapist, considering my issues rather than keeping the focus on their own healing process.

Parents can think along the same lines about disclosures to their children, and about their children's disclosures to the outside world. We have the right to live our lives as we choose, and yes, others should accept those choices if we are not causing harm to others, if we are good and kind, etc. The reality, however, is that certain kinds of families and relationships are considered more socially acceptable than others. No matter what, sharing requires focusing on the positive.

Communication is a two-way street: if you expect your child to tell you about his or her personal explorations, you should expect to occasionally be asked questions in return. That does not, however, mean that you always need to divulge details about your sex life. Disclosure about your own sexual past or preferences in conversations with your child is a very personal decision.

As a psychiatrist, I think about disclosure a lot, both at work and at home. In the old school of Freudian psychoanalysis, we were not supposed to disclose anything about our own lives. Withholding personal information was meant to present the patient with a blank canvas, thus creating the opportunity for transference as the patient made assumptions and "filled in the gaps" with his or her fantasies of the psychiatrist (as friend, lover, parent, teacher, etc.). Modern psychiatric approaches allow for more potential disclosures to help build rapport with the patient. Sharing a bit about your life outside the office, about your partner or children, your hobbies or interests, can be an important part of the process of building trust with a client. In some situations, disclosing information or an identity can foster an alliance. A gay psychiatrist may disclose his sexual orientation to a gay patient if he believes it will make the patient more comfortable, while remaining quiet about his partner choices or the specifics of his sex life.

I believe this also applies to personal disclosures with children. Some disclosures may be useful: "When I was dating, I always started with group dates first so I could get to know the person before being alone with them." Some topics, like talking to teens about the first time you had your heart broken, can be very useful.

Other disclosures, though, may not serve you as well. Think ahead to how your child will process the information. Could telling your teen that you once had an abortion because the relationship was failing be traumatizing to them, causing them to start thinking about their unborn sibling? Disclosing information about how old you were when you lost your virginity, or with whom, or how many sexual partners you have had, is often not helpful because children compare themselves to their parents. Your child may then feel inadequate, uninteresting, or competitive. There are exceptions, of course. The best approach, in my opinion, is to think carefully before you disclose rather than doing so impulsively.

Be especially careful about disclosures of sexual abuse or assault to younger children. If your child was assaulted, it might be appropriate to share your story with the goal of creating mutual empathy, processing, and moving on in a framework of positivity. Just keep in mind that parenting is a pay-it-forward situation, and providing advice and reassurance is the job of a parent to their child. It is best to avoid creating situations where your child is the one who is attempting to provide comfort or reassurance to you.

A Patient's Story: **Ricky**

RICKY IS A 16-YEAR-OLD male who came to see me after his girlfriend, Brie, slapped him during a fight. She was jealous after seeing him with his arm around one of her classmates in an Instagram post. Brie would often lash out at him, hit him, or threaten to harm herself if they argued. When Ricky told his mother what was happening, his mother shared a story of her own with him. She told him that before they were married, Ricky's father had cheated on her and she took an overdose of pills to get his attention.

The story was well-intentioned and had a positive message: his mother realized she had used emotional blackmail, she sought professional help, and the relationship endured. But although Ricky gave his mother a hug and told her that she was very strong, he was disturbed by the story. When we discussed the incident in therapy, Ricky explained that it had upset him to learn that his mother hadn't been mentally stable. He worried that women were "too much trouble" at this stage of his life, or that he could end up hurting someone the way his mother had been hurt, which was worse than he had experienced with Brie.

Instead of telling him such a personal story, Ricky's mother might have said something simpler, like, "If a girl threatens to hurt herself to get you to do something that you don't want to do, that's a red flag. She probably needs professional help, and you'll need to tell her parents, because you aren't equipped to deal with this stuff at your age." She might even have called Brie's parents, depending on the seriousness of the threat.

Avoid oversharing
• • • •

If your child asks you about something that you do not feel comfortable sharing, or if it would not be helpful to provide an honest answer, you can state a boundary rather than tell a lie (no matter how small).

Try saying something like this: "I'm an adult, and would like privacy about things that don't concern you. You'll probably feel the same when you're a parent. I will also respect your privacy as long as I don't believe it affects your safety or well-being. When I became a parent, I signed up to be responsible for those things. So, sometimes I ask questions that I expect you to answer but that I might not answer in return."

Nontraditional families and parent disclosure: one family's story

• • • •

The way that our own sexual story affects our child becomes very clear in the story of Leyla and Samir. Leyla had been married to Samir for more than 30 years when I interviewed her. When he wanted to settle down in their early years, she was torn about whether it was the right decision for her at the time. Here is her account below:

> My reason for choosing nonmonogamy had to do with the fact that I did not ever want to resent Samir for not letting me be single. I've always been in serious relationships, basically since I was 16 years old. I don't think I had a single year that I wasn't dating somebody. When I finally separated from my first husband in San Francisco, all I wanted to do was have the freedom to go where I wanted, to live where I wanted, to do what I wanted to do, and travel wherever I wanted to go. Then, inconveniently, I met Samir. And Samir had absolutely no interest in waiting around until I got my yayas out! He told me, "I may not be around when you come back." And he was absolutely right. He hates being alone and had no interest in staying single. So I had a very tough choice to make–to lose my freedom or to lose a really good guy. But we were so frank with each other, and he ended up doing something that I consider to be one of the most generous acts imaginable. He understood me, and said, "I want you, and I don't want to be in the way of you feeling that freedom." He also told me that he was not that interested in monogamy either, theoretically.

Over the years, their nonmonogamy took different forms, even as their desire to build a marriage "based on absolute honesty and openness and the sharing of literally everything that we might be thinking about sexually" remained constant. When their children were young, Leyla and Samir's outside sexual encounters were infrequent, even though they fantasized about involving others. When they began to experiment, they at first included other men in their sex life together:

> It started with Samir and I being in a threesome, it wasn't me sneaking around. It was more of a kink. Then it evolved into a situation where he was seeing other women and I was seeing other men. Sometimes he would be with us and sometimes he wouldn't, and it wouldn't really matter. What did matter was that if he was not in the room, I had to really fill him in on everything that happened. That shared part of the experience is fundamental to our relationship, and to feeling connected. Those times when I've failed to report back enough, he felt very disconnected and it was damaging to how close we felt to each other.

Most recently, they had both developed polyamorous relationships with other partners that involved much more than sex. Leyla described their current marital relationship as extremely strong and authentic, and as both personally and philosophically fulfilling. Samir, she said, experienced a great deal of "compersion"—or feelings of pleasure while knowing his partner was being pleasured. Beyond the sex, they also both appreciated the other elements that outside partners brought into their lives. She explains:

> I don't really believe that any one person could be everything for their spouse. We can allow each other to be ourselves. Samir loves connecting with women, and has more female than male friends. I'm glad that he has other types of women in his life who can satisfy certain needs he has that I'm not very good at satisfying. And, after 30 years, we're still having so much fun together. We've been allowed to explore, and come back to each other.

Leyla's most recent outside relationship with a lover named Max ended amicably, due to differences in beliefs about parenting. Her lover wanted her to take more of an active role in the lives of his young children, but she was reluctant.

I don't think Max even realizes what it means to ask someone to take on a role as a stepparent of young kids. If you are truly committed to this other person, there is a responsibility to be that person who walks into the room and the kids are happy to see you. It takes an enormous amount of time and work to gain their trust, and if you don't do that, they will see you as that person who takes time with their parent away from them. And then, after you work to become their friend, when they start having medical issues or psychological issues, you can't help but be worried if you're truly integrated. You start going to their school plays, you start worrying about their grades, you start all of that again. So, when he says he needs to be with somebody who is willing to integrate with his family, I don't think he understands how intense that is. It's uncharted water for me, and I don't even want to try again now, because I've been parenting for over 20 years.

Parenting in a nonmonogamous relationship has not always been easy for her. Leyla worries about how her four children, Nadir, Wayne, Omar, and Sophie, have been affected by their parents' choices. In some ways, her relationship with her children had always been very open, to the point where she wondered whether she had tried to be too much of a confidante at times, and too little of a parent. In other ways, however, having an open marriage meant hiding important parts of their lives. Although the children are now aware that their parents are nonmonogamous, that wasn't always the case. In fact, the initial revelation was traumatic–something that she wishes had happened differently. She recounts a story involving her two youngest children:

They learned about our open relationship in a very unfortunate way... A few years ago, I upgraded my laptop and gave my old laptop to Sophie. I deleted my accounts, but forgot to delete a messenger app from the dashboard. She ended up seeing some images there in a message that she shouldn't have seen. When I returned home one day, the kids took me to the kitchen and told me that they wanted to show me something. They pulled out the laptop and showed me the pictures. The pictures weren't ridiculously compromising–I was actually relieved to some extent–but they saw me on a beach, clearly nude, with a man they didn't know. Honestly, it was just like me and the guy took a selfie ... it didn't even show my nipples, but it was definitely obvious that we were lying down with our shirts off. My daughter Sophie was quite young at the time, and very upset. She said, "Who the hell is this man?!"

They thought that I was cheating on Samir and asked if I was going to get a divorce. I told them, "No, I love your dad. We've just been married for a very long time, and sometimes you want to allow yourself to love other people. It's okay with Dad." I can't remember exactly the words that I said ... but they've seen his girlfriends during holidays and parties and things, so I have to believe that they knew some of what was going on. But I had never really fallen in love with any of the guys, while Samir's girlfriends were people that he wanted to integrate into our family life.

So, things became very strained with Sophie, and she was in tears when the subject came up. At one point I said, "Sophie, just imagine that I'm gay. Some people love the same sex, some people love the opposite sex. I'm a person who loves multiple people." But that explanation did not go well; she couldn't handle it. Sophie said, "That's not the same thing." She just thinks our life is absolutely freaky.

Like the other challenges we've faced, that crisis brought my husband and I closer together, because we don't want to repeat mistakes. Eventually, Samir talked with her to help smooth things over. Sophie basically said, "Look, I don't care what you do, but don't shove it down my throat. I don't want to know about it." She feels like it should be handled in a European style–like, just don't talk about it, sweep it under the rug, I don't care, do what you want to do, but I don't want to know about it.

Sophie is under the influence of biased cultural norms around sexuality. She doesn't have as many problems with Samir and the women he sees, yet she seems to think that I'm some kind of a "dirty slut." I also think that Samir is more accepting of a model where the person is integrated into the family, and it's not just physical. In some ways you would think the physical would be less threatening because there would be less interference in our family life. Until recently, I had a boyfriend named Max. It didn't work out with him, but he would have been the one person in the last 30 years that I actually would have considered integrating into our family life. I would have sat down with Sophie and said, "This is real. I just want you to know that he is somebody I really love very much, and I hope you come to like him." But we never got to that point, because Max and I mutually decided to end the relationship.

When Max was around our family over the holidays, I was careful not to show affection to him. All of my sons' cousins and other family members who know are pretty laid-back about everything, but if they had made some sort of comment, I knew things would get worse. Sophie's need to conform and be accepted is unbelievably strong. I'm not even sure she even knows herself well enough to know how she feels about us vis-à-vis what she thinks her friends might think of her because we're her parents. Sometimes, I think she really wants Samir and me to be like other boring suburban–probably miserable–parents. Maybe she will make different choices for herself and live more traditionally. But then I also think that, at the end of the day, when she matures, she'll be able to say, "You two were happy. You had a happy home. You didn't fight. You didn't hurt each other, or try to tear each other to shreds like so many people do. You are loving in your relationships." I think she will come around, but obviously, the process is going to be slow.

With her son Omar, her worries are different.

When your children become teenagers, you start to see a lot of yourself in them, but you don't get to choose what part of yourself. Omar knows that we have an unconventional lifestyle, but I'm not sure he is picking up on the best aspects of it. He's doing well, but I wonder sometimes how he will move into a relationship that grows in a more traditional way. He can't possibly emulate what we are doing at his age. He plays the "hookup" game a lot, pursuing girls... and he talks to girls in a very non-traditional way. But that's only superficially what we do. What we do is so much more profound, because it's about allowing the love of our life to expand through other sexual experiences. I hope that if he chooses to live the way we live, he does so after having a long-term, steady person in his life, because I think that is where you really learn how to be with somebody and how to really empathize with that person. He has expressed his desire to really fall deeply in love with somebody, and I hope that he can have that at least long enough to learn from that connection. Just hooking up is neither good for the girl nor good for him, and it's definitely not the way we are. A big misconception people have of open relationships is that they are totally irresponsible or unaccountable, or that it's a more diffused, sad type of relationship. Actually, I would argue that it is much harder to do what we do than to just remain monogamous and just tolerate each other, but it is rewarding because it is intentional.

Having a proper monogamous relationship as a teen, and really learning what kind of compromises one is willing to make to be close to somebody, is absolutely critical because when you finally have your own kids, you are being inconvenienced all the time! Being in a relationship, half the time is about compromise. Kids who are immature will think that having an open relationship relieves you from the burden of compromise, but that's not true. The kind of relationship we have is about exponential compromise. It's not all about you. That complicates things a lot, even if it's ultimately more rewarding. But I don't think a child, or even a teenager, could really understand that level of effort in our relationship without experiencing those compromises.

Omar and I talk about a lot, though, and I'm open about the things I regret and the things I didn't do right. That's something that I never had with my mother—openness. She was always very defensive. Omar and I have a great relationship now. But with my daughter, Sophie, it's more like living a lie. I guess it's lucky for her that my recent ex, Max, and I are not going to have that kind of serious relationship. Sophie's not going to have to see it. I make an effort to respect her wishes and hide my paramours, for example by talking on the phone with them after she goes to bed and before she gets up. I wish I didn't have to hide from Sophie, but we are not living in a culture where the ideal that I imagine is even possible.

My husband Samir and I love the idea of living in an extended, non-nuclear family structure... If that could be the norm, or even accepted, it would have been easier on the kids. The problem is that there's a difference between what the kids saw around them at home and then when they went to school or to another house for a sleepover, they came home and suddenly saw their family as so different. So if I could live my life again, I'd love to find that simplicity earlier, a situation where other kids have parents doing the same thing and you don't even have to explain it. I'd love it if there was an understanding that those choices are okay, even though not everyone needs to make the same ones. We're so far from that, but if you ask me what I would recommend, I'd recommend that the world change so that parents don't have to be in a position to say why we are different.

I asked her what advice she would give to parents.

You are not going to talk about sex in the same way with a 6-year-old as with a 14-year-old, but it might be prudent to say from a young age that their parents love other people. When they get older, and they're having sex too, if they ask for more details, you can be honest with them without oversharing. You don't talk about things that are not their business, like, "Do you fight with the person?" or "Where does the money come from?" Those kinds of things shouldn't concern them.

Leyla's son Omar spoke with me as well, and he explained that
he initially felt betrayed, but eventually developed a respect for his
parents' choices:

> I realized that some of these people who had been around my
> whole life and joined us on family vacations, maybe they have
> been dating or seeing my parents... It made things a little weird
> and definitely shook up some of my relationships with those
> family friends. Probably former hookups of my parents! So I
> was mistrustful of them for a while because my siblings and I
> felt like we had been lied to. But at the same time, I have never
> really given that much of a crap about how other people lived
> their lives, even my parents. This has been one of my traits—I'm
> pretty open to different people living their lives in different ways.
> I see value in a lot of different lifestyles, not necessarily just ones
> reflective of my own. My parents taught me that we are a differ-
> ent family and we can't compare ourselves with other families.

Omar admitted that coming to terms with his parents' open marriage had influenced his own views on relationships, but that it was
a positive influence.

> I've always been really cynical about marriage. I grew up in San
> Francisco, where half of my friends' parents were divorced! So
> I've always been cynical and I've never been religious. I think I
> always kind of understood how difficult relationships are. It's
> just a statistical rarity that your marriage will be successful for
> the rest of your life. What my parents have done is find a really
> interesting solution to a problem that is often based in sexual
> frustration. I would love to have a similar relationship with my
> future partner. I feel having an open relationship is unprece-
> dented when you are young (which explains why most of us just
> pursue no-strings hookups instead). I would prefer an open rela-
> tionship. It'd be really nice for the high school years, because
> then I could gain more emotional support in my life. I could
> really use that in high school, which is a landscape of insecurities.

Leyla responded to Omar's comments:

What concerns me about Omar's relationships is his lack of connection with these young women. He has sex with lots of different young women, but he fails to connect or fall in love. I worry that his parents' narrative has prevented him from trying out monogamy even short-term, as he has not seen it as a model.

Omar's response:

I don't see the point of dating unless someone is ready to be serious. There is a halt of progression and there is a lot to do in the high school/college years. High school and college days are such a shit show for dating, and it's not just a sexist judgment but a reality of my environment. It's just like, the way our society views females creates more conformist girls, and it's not until later in their life when they realize that everything they have been following their whole lives is total bullshit and they should really find their own narrative.

So Omar feels that most of the girls in his school were afraid to be different and wanted to conform, but he didn't feel that pressure. As for the boys, he said,

Males are equally guilty of this adherence to the gendered narrative—it's more accepted in our culture for males to behave like "dogs" AND be successful, smart, and more cutting-edge than females. Due to everyone in high school following these false narratives, I feel there are a lot of fake people you are surrounded by in high school. Being real comes later in life. So, later in life is when I will be able to have genuine connections with people.

Although Leyla and Samir are an example of a couple who are willing to experiment with nonmonogamy and family arrangements that we could call nontraditional, your sexual story and what you choose to disclose always affects your child—even if your story is extremely traditional. The types of options that your child can imagine for themselves in the future, the things that excite them or that they fear, the things they want in a partner or for themselves–these are all heavily influenced by you and your story.

Blender, banner, & chameleon: family disclosures to the world

• • • •

Nontraditional families may face more scrutiny and unique challenges, but all parents will occasionally need to consider how their own sexuality will impact their child, not just in terms of their relationship, but also socially. How you choose to disclose your preferences to the outside world can be very tough for many families. Some are more open, which I call "banner," some try to blend in, which I call "blender" or "in the closet," and the mix of the two is "chameleon." Do not forget to consider the repercussions of disclosures for your child as well as for yourself. It is essential to remember that while you may have consciously chosen your politics or your lifestyle, your child did not. Considering your child's needs for privacy with teachers or peers is essential to building trust and respect. During the early years, children are not aware of all the nuances of social interactions; it is somewhat easier for parents to control the flow of information to the outside world.

Children raised in same-sex or polyamorous families, for instance, often do not recognize that their family is different from others' during the early years. As children are egocentric at young ages, they don't really think to compare themselves to others. Dr. Elisabeth Sheff has studied polyamorous families and is considered an expert in this field. According to her research and her book *The Polyamorists Next Door*, some of the children she interviewed expressed gratitude at having more parental figures in their life to give them attention.

Still, children may go through phases (especially as they approach their teen years) where they want total discretion from you, or privacy with certain friends or within certain environments. One hallmark of being a teenager is the desire to blend in with one's peers. Any sign of being different is interpreted as embarrassing. Unfortunately, some children may face bullying or are ostracized for their parents' choices. The teens themselves may go through waves of being more and less comfortable with their family's choices.

A Human Story: Gabbi

GABBI AND HER SAME-SEX partner are currently raising their children in Arkansas. She was surprised when their youngest daughter, Anna, was reluctant to schedule a playdate with a new friend from school. When one of her moms questioned her about it, Anna said, "Sometimes I just want to be a normal family. When you kiss, I get embarrassed." Although they initially did not want to hide their relationship, they decided to compromise in the beginning. When the new friend came over, only one of the moms was home, to avoid questions being raised about who the other woman was. But after the child had visited a few times, she told Anna, "Your mom is cool." They introduced the second mom, and the rest of the relationship flowed smoothly. Even later, the other child continued to make comments like, "It's fun you have two moms to go shopping with!" As trust was built in the friendship and over time, everyone was able to be themselves.

Blender families

In my practice, as mentioned above, I see three general types of families with regard to how they present themselves to the outside world: blender, banner, and chameleon. Blender families are "in the closet" about their family structure. They may be gay or polyamorous, but they believe that their community is not accepting of their choices. These families try to blend in, disguising partners who do not conform to the mainstream. Sometimes the other partner is presented as a friend, roommate, or relative. Blending in makes it easier for families to participate in community life without having to explain their personal arrangements. Although this may make certain aspects of social life easier, it can also leave the nonnormative partner feeling left out and unable to take a validated role in child care.

A Human Story: Bob and Tanya

A COUPLE WHOM I had the pleasure of interviewing, Bob and Tanya, live in a Mormon community in Idaho and raise Bob's three children from his previous marriage. Their ages are 12, 14, and 17. For the last six years, Bob has been dating a new partner, Gary, exclusively. Tanya is aware of and supports the relationship, and cares for Gary as a very good friend. Bob and Tanya have agreed that they would rather stay together as a unit. Rather than get divorced, they have decided to "rent a room" to Gary so that he can live with them while the family's privacy is maintained. Tanya has had affairs, although she chooses lovers from outside the community and never introduces them to the children. In their conservative community, this is perhaps the most comfortable strategy, at least while the children are living at home. Understandably, however, it leaves Gary with mixed emotions about whether his contributions to the household as a partner and co-parent are recognized.

Banner families

Banner families are families that do not try to hide their differences from the mainstream, and sometimes even take a political stance in the community. Some polyamorous couples, for example, introduce their lovers to their children or work colleagues as girlfriend/boyfriend or partner. Poly or same-sex parents may be involved at local gay and lesbian centers, march in parades, or mentor other individuals in the community. I love following @daddyandpapa on Instagram: they are a same-sex male couple with two adorable children of mixed race. One of the men is an army veteran, and the family travels around the country in an Airstream with the agenda of breaking stereotypes. They call the goal of their actions "acceptance through visibility."

Although some children adapt readily to such an approach to the outside world, others find themselves at odds with their parents' beliefs or practices.

A Human Story: **Stella and Rob**

STELLA AND ROB live in Houston with their two children, Jenny (aged nine) and Claire (aged four). When they initially decided to open up their marriage, they kept the decision secret from friends and family. Over time, however, Stella started dating other partners more seriously. They began opening up in their community, even speaking in a documentary about their arrangement. Being a banner family posed challenges. One of the most painful experiences Stella had was when her own brother refused to speak to her for a year. Although friends reassured her that he would eventually come around, this was not a great consolation for Stella.

Their family evolved, and when Stella found a new partner named Jacob, they began living in a large compound including multiple homes. Stella's husband Rob began dating Sally, a woman with an

11-year-old son. Stella and her new partner Jacob became primary partners, and had a son together. Stella and Rob's two children, Jenny and Claire, love their new little brother, and are always holding him in their family photos. The entire family is open on social media, and sends out Christmas cards each year.

Living so openly takes courage, and I have been happily amazed at the support they have received from their community and within their own family. Jenny and Claire love their stepbrother from Jacob's previous marriage and their new half-brother that Jacob and their mother have had, and are thriving under the care of four parental figures. I have seen no evidence of any trauma from their kibbutz-like arrangement, although all of the parents are carefully considering how best to maneuver through the necessary transitions of adolescence and the high school years.

Because the partners in the above example share values, and remain good friends with each other, communication is open and regular. In the case of a contentious divorce, or other situations where sets of parental figures choose fundamentally different lifestyles, serious fighting can ensue. Children will unfortunately be caught in the middle of such battles, suffering trauma when parents cannot overcome their differences. Being a banner family will take an additional toll under these circumstances, as their openness could be leveraged against them and misinterpreted in the courts.

Chameleon families

Chameleon families mix blender and banner styles. They may be open in some situations and with some people, while using varying degrees of discretion in other situations and with other people. Both parents and children may take care to appear mainstream when at work or school, for example, or with certain relatives.

A Human Story: Nina

I INTERVIEWED NINA, who is in a relationship triad composed of three women: Nina, Alexandra, and Sarah. Nina is the birth mother, Alexandra is her wife, and Sarah is their third partner. Together they raise their children. They live in an open-minded community in Chicago, and are privileged to mostly be able to be out about their arrangement. Yet, because their oldest daughter Grace is undergoing a difficult period in her own development, including coming to terms with her own sexual identity, she does not always want to explain her family to her peers. The women are understanding, and Grace plays a role in the decision-making process about when they will be "out" and when they will be on the "down low."

Nina says:

When children are born, they are born with their own personality, and for some kids, understanding their family is going to be possible and easy, and for other kids it's going to be impossible or very difficult. We have four kids to train between the three of us [female triad], and each one of them handled it in a completely different way.

We've tried to figure out what they need with their different friends. Our oldest, Grace, is 13, and she has some friends that she is out to and others she is not. She was actually fine until she was about 9 or 10, and then one day on a school bus field trip she said, "Look, there is Sarah's apartment!" And someone said, "Who is Sarah?" and she said, "My mom's girlfriend." And then the friend said, "I thought your mom was married?" Until that day, she was totally out there with everything. But that's when it hit her, and she kind of went back into the closet with it. Some friends she will invite out with us, but she'll say, "You guys have to show a lot of discretion. This person doesn't know about it, and I don't want you all touching or kissing or anything." With other friends, she doesn't care. I think it's hard on her, honestly. We try to be sensitive to what she needs. She is fine with Sarah coming to pick her up after school, even though she's not her parent. Sarah goes to all the brunches and those things. Sarah is like the trusted family friend in that context.

We don't pretend that we are not poly, but we can show some discretion for a couple hours and it's not the end of the world. The other thing is making sure that children understand that these are consenting adults. If you hide stuff, then it makes it seem like you are doing something that's bad or that you are not proud of, and then you have second-guessing on everything else that's going on. So I think it's really important not to hide it from the kids.

Even siblings may come to different resolutions with their parents' decisions. For example, in the story of Leyla and Samir, the couple with the open marriage whose two youngest children discovered compromising photos on their mother's old laptop, Omar and Sophie found out as teens that their parents were intentionally nonmonogamous, and Omar was able to come to terms with it by taking a banner approach once he got used to the idea: "My parents are strange, but they do their own thing and all of my friends and I accept it."

Omar's younger sister Sophie, on the other hand, remained ashamed of her parents and embarrassed in front of her friends. She often stated that her parents were "gross," and didn't want to invite friends over to the house. Her mother received the brunt of her anger. When asked about the mistakes of her parents, Sophie said, "I already felt so different from other people that it impeded me from making connections with other kids, and I had surface connections."

Community and location matter too. A same-sex couple raising their children in New York sought out a church community. They got recommendations from lesbian friends and eventually found a

Catholic church where their family was accepted. This might not have been possible in less progressive communities.

Although Omar, the 18-year-old son of Leyla and Samir, sometimes wished that his parents had been forthcoming with him earlier about their open marriage, he also recognized that, as a preteen and teenager, he would have wanted community support (you can read more about Omar's story from his perspective on page 181).

Omar's parents could have sought out local polyamory groups in their community to make connections for the kids. Sometimes, meeting similar types of families can be helpful. Even so, though, teen angst could still arise around a parent's choices.

Families can change their approach depending on the circumstances, over time, or with certain people. Compromise does not necessarily mean bowing to shame and censure; it can be more of a way to allow everyone in the family an opportunity to interact with the outside world in a way that feels comfortable and authentic.

There is still a fear of stigma and rejection that includes discrimination at work, rejection from family members, and custody issues. Polyamorous families still struggle with assumptions that they are sex addicts or perverts, and thus cannot be good parents. They may also worry about the legal repercussions of their choices.

To disclose or not to disclose
• • • •

Diana Adams, a well-respected mediator, family lawyer, and advocate for nontraditional families, told me in an interview:

> I talk with many parents about setting appropriate boundaries and about how we can be sex-positive parents who do not shame children about sexuality, but also do not place children at odds with the greater society. I often suggest that it is inappropriate for children to keep secrets for adults. So, you need to think about the greater ramifications of any disclosures to your children. You need to think about what your child might say to others...

Sex-positive parents can really be under attack, so it's worth thinking about how to pass on the ideas and values you want to convey to your child while also considering what's going to be safe for them to express in a larger, more sex-negative culture.

Maria Pallotta-Chiarolli, a founding member of the Australian GLBTIQ Multicultural Council, describes these families as "Border Families." She writes, "There needs to be a discursive shift to models of diversity and multiplicity that erase constructs of Center and Margin and that incorporate all families and sexualities. Instead of problematizing and pathologizing certain families and sexualities, there is a need to problematize their problematization and pathologization."

9

Parental
Conflict

● ● ● ●

WHERE I SEE parents doing the most psychological damage to their children is in how they handle parental conflict. This also affects the children's romantic relationships in the future. I see dozens of patients come into my office talking about their fear of trusting or commitment in relationship. Due to their parents, they saw ugly separation and divorce. When things are not working out, no matter what kind of relationship you are in, it's not the divorce itself but the way you break up that really matters. This chapter will help parents think through these issues.

Divorce
· · · ·

The trickiest part of divorce is explaining to children why romantic love has ended. Children often think it might be their fault, so reassuring them that it's not is critical. You can explain that the romantic love has ended. "Romantic love is when two people find each other and sometimes get married and make a baby like you." You can add, "When two people are in romantic love, they often have sex and decide to make a baby like in your case" (this can be modified depending on family structure). "Sometimes romantic love ends, like for us. We were not getting along all of the time, and felt we would be happier living apart. But this had nothing to do with what you did, and you are not to blame. We still have family love, which is a powerful bond that will live on because we love you."

Remember that your children's issues may not be the same as yours; they may be more concerned about what their new bedroom will look like rather than how much time they will spend at which parent's house. Children may identify with one parent more than the other (a daughter may identify more with her mother during the separation or divorce). This is normal, but it is not always healthy. If your child does not want to spend time at the other parent's home, that does not mean this is best. They should be encouraged to divide up their time in a healthy way–or else parental alienation may ensue.

"Parental alienation" is a term that means a child being forced to choose sides between the parents. One parent may set up a framework that makes it difficult for a child to spend time with the other parent, by using directly hostile or passive-aggressive measures. For example, one parent may seek to make a child feel guilty for wanting to spend time with the other parent by being needy or placing the child in the parentified role. This could involve saying something like, "If you leave me this weekend, I will be lonely, as I have no one else who loves me" (passive-aggressive). It can also be expressed in openly hostile terms: "You know what he said to me, he is a liar." You can NEVER speak badly of the other parent, and if you do, you should apologize immediately. Also take care that your child doesn't hear you when you are talking to family members or friends about the other parent. These situations can do a lot of damage not only to the family structure but to psychological well-being, and may result in long-term parental estrangement.

Don't use your child as a spy

In any family situation where a child moves between households, it is important that parents do not criticize each other in front of the child. Constant conflict can affect your child's health and well-being. Parents must also resist the temptation to interrogate a child for information about the other parent or other household. Your child is not a spy. Give the other parent their privacy. If you feel there is a real issue to be addressed, then address it with your former partner. But seeking problems will inevitably lead to more problems. When children are used as spies or weapons, they can develop emotional issues, depression, guilt, and anger disorders.

Divorce in nontraditional families

No matter what your family structure, divorce is very tricky. It is even trickier for those in nontraditional families. Diana Adams explains that in divorce cases where one parent has been in a nontraditional relationship, the judge has often sided with the birth parent who is single over a birth parent in a nontraditional relationship even if both parents are honest, hardworking people. "There's a history of single moms being accused of being sex addicts," Adams said when I interviewed her, "and having that used against them in child custody cases. Now that's extended to people who are polyamorous, or kinky. We don't have enough research yet to support those people in a courtroom setting and demonstrate that their family or relationship structure falls within the realm of healthy, adult sexual expression."

Given that more than half of marriages end up in divorce, and that many single people date and have sex with more than one person at a time, polyamory does not seem like sexual deviancy to me. Being polyamorous also does not mean that parents would expose their children to inappropriate behavior. Many teens are polyamorous, whether or not they call it such. They may say they are looking for "the one"–a healthy monogamous relationship–but then take a "friends with benefits" approach to sex because they do not want to settle down at a young age.

Children born into polyamorous families may not consider themselves polyamorous, for a variety of reasons, including the desire for cultural acceptance. Parents can try to send a message of acceptance and of being "true to the moment"; people's desires can change over the life course, and what we want at 17 is not necessarily what we want at 37 or 50. And open relationships are not for everyone, regardless of age. It is important for teens to know that the kind of relationship their polyamorous parents have may not be possible for them for many years. Sometimes, at the beginning of a relationship, partners are not open to sharing. There are biological reasons for this, such as the release of oxytocin, serotonin, and dopamine that accompanies sexual activity and creates bonding between partners. There are also emotional reasons, such as the need to feel secure as a couple before opening up to others.

Disclosing infidelity

Infidelity is a tricky parenting issue, because regardless of anyone's reasons for cheating, lying and betrayal are still behaviors that most parents would never condone. Children may feel the need to take sides against the parent who has engaged in the infidelity, and although this may be somewhat gratifying to the betrayed partner, it is best to try to avoid such a situation. Children always identify with both parents, regardless of who is to blame. Talking negatively about a partner can sometimes backfire.

Infidelity does not arise in a bubble, and there are always two sides to every story—two sides that are probably too complex to explain to a young child and perhaps inappropriate even in the teen years. Setting up a betrayer/victim dynamic can be detrimental. A child who sees one parent vilified by the other parent can become afraid of losing the parent altogether. Explaining that mistakes were made but that no one is to blame can be important *and* mature. You may have your own opinions about the matter, but remember: *it has nothing to do with your child*.

In situations of emotional or physical betrayal, a child can again be put into a caretaking role. Even if you have experienced something traumatic, it is important not to forget that the experience is traumatic for your child as well. Some children may identify with the pain of the hurt party (mother/father/same-sex couple—the rules still apply). Another child may take the stance of a diplomat, staying out of it and saying, "This is not my business." Sometimes children are even angrier when they are older.

Reassure your child that no matter how angry you might be at the other parent, the child has done nothing wrong. As well, try to control your emotions in front of the child, because you may be able to end the marriage, but you will need to maintain the positive parental relationship regardless of the circumstances. If your child does see you cry, speak harshly, or act out in anger, acknowledge the emotion and move on: "I was angry, but we will get through it."

Moving between households

· · · ·

Some children need to move between households due to a divorce or other situations. Children are smart enough to understand that different rules hold in each family, and that they must adapt to each environment. Here are some amazing tips on how to make this happen.

My house, my rules

Divorced parents often complain to me, "We need to get on the same page in terms of household rules," but this is simply a misconception. Rules should be consistent *within* each household, not *between* them. Children easily adapt to the need for different behaviors in different settings.

Parents must try to respect the fact that each household may have unique rules. If a child is struggling behaviorally or in school, they unfortunately sometimes blame the other parent or suggest that rules are not being uniformly enforced. While children adapt to different settings with different rules, what is more difficult for them is dealing with conflict between households.

Create space for your child

In each household, children should be given their own space. Allowing them to pick the paint color for the walls, the sheets for the bed, and which items will decorate the room gives them a sense of ownership. If your child has treasured items, such as special blankies or favorite toys, you might want to purchase one for each home so that they do not feel they need to choose.

Parents worry about things that don't really matter to children, such as whether the size of the bedroom is the same or if one of the parents has a pool, a bigger yard, or a nicer car. What matters most to children is whether their parents are happy and kind to them—and, especially, that they are not asked to choose between the parents or play favorites. It is also important for parents to meet their child's expectations by picking them up from school when promised, getting them to bed on time, or following through on social obligations. Bedtimes might be different in each house, but each household should be consistent in enforcing its own rules. One of the young girls in my practice, Clarissa, has a bedtime of 7:30 p.m. at her mother's house, where she has her own room. At her father's house, she shares a bedroom with her older brother, Jimmy, and to make things easier, both siblings are allowed to stay up until 9:30. Clarissa is fine with both arrangements.

Dealing with an ex's new partner and parental arrangements

• • • •

Although we choose our own intimate partners, we do not get to choose those of our previous partners when they form new relationships. You may feel nervous that the new stepparent will not share your values, turn your child's birth parent against you, or steal your child's affection. I encourage worried parents to try to put their jealousy aside and give the new partner the benefit of the doubt.

A Patient's Story: Garett

GARETT WAS A 12-year-old boy in my practice whose parents were divorcing due to multiple affairs and betrayals. The parents refused to speak to each other, and at one point his father, Len, claimed that Garett's mother, Janet, was "a stranger" to him. When Len's girlfriend became pregnant, they did not tell Garett. Instead, Garett's mother, Janet, noticed the girlfriend's burgeoning belly during one of their drop-offs and asked Garett about it. Garett was confused, and then asked his father about it on the next visit. Not wanting to give Janet any information about his life, Len denied that his girlfriend was pregnant. Garett's confusion grew. After the child was born, Len told Garett about his new brother. The whole situation backfired, as Garett not only felt as though he was being replaced but also believed that his father could not be trusted. Garett became very insecure about his place in the family, having panic attacks at school and complaining of suicidal thoughts.

Garett struggled with these feelings and his father, who felt he was acting in his son's best interest by protecting him, did not agree with the view of taking a more collaborative approach. I ended up referring Garett to a male therapist, as I felt that he needed an appropriate, loving, and honest male role model. This was greatly beneficial to Garett, and through the relationship with his new male therapist he was able to work through his depression and foster better relationships in school.

More is more

I remind parents in this situation that having another parent can be an incredible asset to a child. Giving the stepparent the benefit of the doubt alleviates some of the stress involved in taking on such a role. Talking openly about your values, and what you hope the person can offer your child, is also beneficial. Empower the stepparent to develop a close relationship with your child. Allow them to spend time alone or pursue shared interests. Give this new partner permission to do with the child the things they are best at. For example, if the new partner is a firefighter, maybe he could take your child on a tour of the firehouse.

The stepparent can never replace you, or pose a threat to the love your child has for you. Allowing your child to develop bonds with other adults can be healthy for all of you. (And maybe you'll even enjoy having some personal time for yourself!)

Let go

Maintaining a personal stance that is open both to change and to letting go of the need for control will help you balance your emotions. Keeping some distance both practically and emotionally will also allow the other parents to do their job in their own unique way. Of course, some people are not fit to be parents, such as drug addicts or people with serious mental health problems. If this is truly the case, then it may be necessary to intervene. However, in the majority of cases I have seen, the stepparents are good people who are caught up in the jealous struggles or control battles of the birth parents. These stepparents are not trying to take over, but truly want what is best for the children. They may even be in a unique place to see what is best, given that they do not have the emotional history with the other birth parent that their partner does. A stepparent could be an asset in intervening where either birth parent is not behaving in the best interests of the child.

All parents will make mistakes. If a stepparent makes a decision you do not like, and that is not life-threatening, let it go. I mean it: *let it go*.

If you must say something, do so in a constructive way. Most of these situations can be likened to a dad changing a diaper for the first time. That dad is not going to kill the child by putting the diaper on backwards. Yes, the feces will run all over the place. It will be a mess. But he will eventually figure it out before the child is toilet trained or after he gets his second shirt stained. If you chastise a parent for such a mistake, they may avoid ever stepping up again. And then what have you gained? A marginalized and disempowered parent, knee-deep in shit, and more diaper changing for yourself.

Try to approach stepparents the same way. You may not be overjoyed that your ex's new spouse took your child to McDonald's, forgetting about their low-sugar diet. But one Happy Meal is not the end of the world, is it? And it is definitely not worth the fight if, after McDonald's, they went to a batting park and had an amazing time while you got your nails done and went to the gym. Stepparents can be a win-win.

Dating & introducing new partners

• • • •

One of the biggest struggles for single parents comes with dating. Questions I often get asked are:

- How do I describe my new partner? (*"Do I call them 'my friend' or 'my girlfriend'?"*)

- When is it appropriate to introduce my new partner to my children?

- Should I be honest that this is a new relationship, which may or may not work out?

- Do I wait until I am certain that this relationship will withstand the test of time even though it has been a few months and we are getting serious?

Deciding how to handle dating situations can be an issue in any relationship, and there are pros and cons to any approach. For example:

- **PRO:** It is often difficult to hide the fact that you are dating someone new, and child care is expensive and not always practical.

- **CON:** Bringing another adult into your child's life can lead to emotional attachments.

- **PRO:** There are benefits to having adult role models outside the family, especially for single parents.

- **CON:** There are also risks. A breakup not only affects you, it also impacts your child.

A Patient's Story: **Barry**

BARRY WAS AN EIGHT-YEAR-OLD boy in my practice who found out by surprise that his father was dating a new woman. His father called him the night before picking him up for the weekend and told him that there would be a "nice lady" in the house when he got there. Barry's parents did not live together but had occasionally discussed getting back together, and had reignited their romance, even though they were still divorced and living separately. They also had game nights and dinners together, which Barry enjoyed. When he got home from the weekend, he was visibly upset. He told his mother that he had been replaced by a new woman who was in his dad's house, because she sat in his favorite chair at the dinner table and stayed overnight in his dad's room. Essentially, he was upset that "now there is this new woman, she sat in my chair... she was nice, but she was not like my mom."

When Barry told his mother about the girlfriend, his mother was furious, as she did not know that her own romantic relationship with Barry's father had ended. A fight erupted between Barry's parents, which he witnessed. The amicable separation was no longer peaceful and both parties lawyered up. Barry then became a mediator between the parents, and started acting out in school and at home. Instead of getting angry at his father for having a new relationship, Barry became angry with his mother and began to hit her. He couldn't even explain why he was so angry at his mother, when it was his father whose actions had caused the conflict. This made his mother feel doubly victimized—first by Barry's father, and then by her son.

Introductions are best done in stages and in a neutral environment, not after a new partner has already moved into the house, and children should never be placed in the role of being the messenger to the other parent. If you've already put your child in this position, it might be a good idea to sit down with them as soon as you can and apologize for it. Explain that you made a mistake by not telling their other parent yourself.

Suggested ideas for introducing new partners

More and more often, modern families need to adapt to new constellations of family members. Having another parental figure around is mostly a great thing. Following some simple guidelines for the introduction of a new partner will make it easier for your child to be accepting of the new normal in your home.

1   **Make sure a relationship has a good possibility of lasting before bringing your child into the equation.** You can evade questions from your child about dating until you are sure that your partner is the right fit for you, is of sound mind, and is ready to take on some sort of parenting role. If they end up meeting the person before you've had a chance to decide whether your new partner is in it for the long haul (because these things happen), introducing that person as a "friend" might be a white lie, but it will be understandable later when you explain your reasoning. Although I would not recommend lying to your child if they ask you directly, "Are you dating?" or "Are you having sex with that person?" I think it is better to say something like, "That's really not something you need to worry about," or "I am entitled to my privacy when it comes to my sex life. I'll let you know if I am dating someone who is serious enough that it would affect you." This is preferable to lying, as children are often astute and it might impact your child's ability to trust you if they find out the truth.

2   **Do not bring your child into your dating life.** The biggest problem that I see arise in single parenting is switching roles. If a parent

starts asking the child about what they should wear on a date, or reporting back on how a date went, the child is thrust into the role of friend or parent. Not only does this undermine the parent's authority, it can be very confusing for the child.

3 **Children should never be placed in the role of being the messenger to the other parent.** Family attorney Diana Adams states that this "messenger" situation is one of the main reasons people end up in costly court battles. I have witnessed this firsthand and I agree: it is always a disaster! Maintaining honesty with the other parent, even if communications are kept brief, is always better.

4 **Introduce a new partner in stages, in neutral territory, and ideally during a structured activity.** When it is time to introduce a new partner to your child, plan a fun activity like ice skating or visiting the zoo, where everyone can be involved. The time frame should be limited, allowing the child time to process afterwards.

5 **Take care to give your child a sense of control over the situation.** When meetings take place in the home, it is important not to disrupt routines and rituals, but to allow the child to be part of the introduction. For example, the new partner might ask the child where they should sit, or inquire about the child's favorite activities.

6 **Most importantly, do not make the introduction during a time of crisis or emotional turmoil.** Such times would include right after you announce the divorce, or during their final exams, etc. It is important that your child not be in a state of trauma when you layer on more drama. This will have the opposite effect, and may cause more damage for them to endure.

Stepparenting tips

• • • •

Stepparents often worry about stepping on the toes of the birth parent. I frequently get questions about how involved stepparents should be in raising the children. Having more than two parents, in my opinion, can be beneficial. The more attention and care a child receives, the better off they will be.

Ideally, stepparents and birth parents should discuss their parenting approach in detail, including both philosophical issues, such as which values to impart, and practical issues, such as how to handle chores or discipline. A big one to make sure you align on is sex education. If you are the stepparent and your stepchild approaches you directly with questions about sex, you might refer them back to the birth parent before answering–unless you've already discussed how to handle such situations. But a stepparent can be a great asset to your child, perhaps appearing as someone more approachable for certain types of questions. Once permission has been obtained from both birth parents, I think the stepparent could be a great resource for the child.

In my practice, I see more parents who do not want the obligations of child rearing than parents who try to shoulder the entire load. So, when I see a parent–whether biological, polyamorous, step, adoptive, or otherwise–who is willing to step up and genuinely participate in a relationship in the best interests of the child, I want to encourage cooperation and an open-minded attitude towards the possibilities.

10

Boost & Embolden Self-Esteem in Your Child

• • • •

JUST AS REGULAR WORKOUTS are important for building physical strength, positive thinking and stress reduction practices should be part of a daily routine to build your child's self-esteem. Eating well, getting good sleep, and exercising are also critical practices for developing self-esteem.

Feed them well
• • • •

Encouraging your child to focus on healthy eating will help them to maintain a good weight, have pleasant-smelling breath, and feel great from the inside out. I encourage parents to adopt at least part of the "slow food" movement within the family. Finding local and organic food sources, avoiding packaged foods and fast-food restaurants, and staying mindful when eating are all beneficial practices. In addition to healthy eating, parents, you might want to try a supplement called L-5-methyltetrahydrofolate, which helps with anxiety and depression and is found in Thorne prenatal vitamins, which is a brand I like (and it works for males too!). Also, fish oil–one gram of EPA DHA from small fish sources such as those offered by Nordic Naturals–can help with focus and concentration.

Help them rest well
• • • •

Sleeping well is essential to mental health and body-positive self-esteem. Sleep training from an early age is essential. Young children should sleep in their own bed, free from light and noise. If you experience difficulties, there are many books on the subject. Older children should also practice good sleeping habits: turning off screens and TV an hour before bedtime, no blue light; no caffeine after noon; using the bed only for sleeping and not for homework, television, or playing video games; getting up and going to bed at the same times each day; and using relaxation techniques when they have difficulty sleeping.

For kids who still have trouble falling or staying asleep, try binaural beats meditation. Binaural beats is a form of music that has an underlying beat mimicking the brainwaves emitted during sleep. This consistent rhythmic sound has a powerful sleep-inducing effect. Ancient/Tribal peoples have used this beat to induce a trancelike meditative state, and we can use it to our advantage to help children fall asleep naturally. There are many examples of this online if you want to look it up; you can also purchase binaural tracks, and these can really help relax the mind. You can also find free videos on YouTube or choose from a variety of mobile applications (just be sure that your child is not giving in to the temptation to keep checking their phone, which will keep them awake!). Children over the age of five can take a three-milligram dose of melatonin for occasional insomnia or for help with jet lag, and you can find this herbal supplement in chewable form in most drugstores or health food stores.

Get them moving
• • • •

Exercising is essential for all children. Sports, gym class, and yoga are great ways to help with anxiety. Very short, intense exercise–like running around the outside of the house as fast as you can–can be a great way to handle anger or anxiety because it will bring the heart rate up and calm the body down. In larger cities there are often free or low-cost recreation centers, which offer swimming pools and athletic programs for kids of all ages.

Practice radical self-acceptance
• • • •

This technique also helps develop one's self-esteem by promoting an understanding of ourselves as the sum of our lives, constantly growing. Radical self-acceptance is a Buddhist principle used by Dr. Marsha Linehan in dialectical behavior therapy (DBT)–what I keep referring to as "Buddha therapy" for the sake of distilling the principles for this book. Radical self-acceptance can help your children manage their thoughts and their self-esteem.

The word "dialectical" means "concerned or acting with opposing forces." In the context of Buddha therapy, it is the balance between change and acceptance. The Serenity prayer is a great example of the practice of radical self-acceptance: "Grant me the serenity to accept the things I cannot change, the courage to change the things I can, and the wisdom to know the difference." Your teenager can accept themselves for their flaws and weaknesses, but also want to change things about themselves that they have power over. This is the balance between change and acceptance.

You can also explain to your teen that the present moment doesn't just leap into being, but is shaped by the millions of things that have happened to you in your life. It's easy to blame yourself or get down on yourself if you think of all the poor decisions you have made or every failure you have had. Many of the bad things that have happened are out of your control, and when you recognize this, it is easier to let go of the need to blame yourself or others. If your teen has a fight with a friend, for example, the fight doesn't need to be interpreted as something that suddenly emerged. The roots of the misunderstanding grew long before. A breakup might have to do with one partner's need for independence, and not be in any way the fault of the other.

Acceptance allows us to feel our emotions without trying to judge the situation or pull away from the other people involved. This does not mean that we put up with mistreatment from others. Rather, it is an inner process of accepting our actual, present-moment experience. It means feeling sorrow and pain without resisting. It means feeling desire or dislike for something or someone without judging the feeling, or feeling compelled to act. Acceptance allows you to be present in your sadness or anger without running away, or being *so* "blinded by rage" that you can't see the obvious.

Practice meditating early on

• • • •

Meditation is known to promote health and well-being, and the medical community is beginning to recognize the benefits. When most people think of meditation, the first thing that comes to mind is seated meditation practices, where an individual is trying to clear their mind, but in fact meditation can take a variety of forms. Guided visual meditations and easy breathing exercises may be much easier for children to understand and practice. Research suggests there are positive impacts of meditation in reducing stress and enhancing general well-being. Meditation may also be helpful for the treatment of anxiety, addiction, aggression, suicidality, and depression.

Start early with your child to develop a meditation practice. Just 10 minutes at the beginning or the end of the day can help everyone in the family learn how to manage stress and better understand their emotions. You may be skeptical, but try it and see how you feel.

I like using apps with the teenagers I work with, such as Headspace and Calm, and often use the apps within sessions to work on concepts. I think parents and teenagers can do these apps together at bedtime or in the morning as a family. This might be a way for the whole family to bond over the experience.

Don't feel bad about offering age-appropriate rewards to your child as a way of encouraging them to continue the practice—and you might need to reward yourself as well!

Don't think that things need to be perfect to meditate—you're seated on a cushion, mind perfectly clear, incense lit, and so on. If everything needs to be perfect, you might never find the time. But you can meditate in the grocery line by focusing on your breathing, your body, being present and aware. Meditation can become a positive habit and part of your daily routine over time.

Breathe. Relax.
· · · ·

Breathing is something that we do naturally, unconsciously. However, it is also something that we can train ourselves to do more efficiently. Our breathing can affect our posture, our psychological state, and our overall health. Correct breathing can stimulate the vagus nerve, which can make you feel more relaxed and control stress hormones that cause anxiety. Athletes use different styles of breathing to enhance their performance. A weightlifter, for example, may inhale and hold to increase her strength and stability. A long-distance runner, though, would need to settle into a rhythmic pattern. Our breath, combined with certain movements, can even be used to control pain. A nurse might ask a patient to inhale before an injection but coach a woman in labor to push during each controlled exhale.

Sometimes we get in the habit of breathing too shallowly or quickly. To begin the breathing exercise, first try a sitting position on the floor. Put one or two hands on your lower abdomen and practice watching your or your child's belly expand on the inhale and contract on the exhale. Most children do the opposite, and it will require some retraining to change this habit.

Alternate nostril breathing: After breathing deeply a few times, hold your ring finger against one of your nostrils (if you use your index finger, you may push too hard). Then inhale slowly through the other nostril, filling your lungs to capacity. Switch to your other hand and nostril, and exhale slowly. Repeat an even number of times on each side.

Square breathing: This exercise is easy to learn but requires some mental effort—meaning that it can distract you when emotions are running high. Breathe in and count to five. Breathe out and hold to five. Continue in repetitions of four (in, out; in, out).

Give yourself and your kids a TIPP

• • • •

Coping with overwhelming emotions is as easy as TIPP. TIPP skills were first taught in Buddha therapy. Remember DBT by Dr. Linehan? Her work is so helpful with teenagers. I use these simple techniques to produce amazing results. When a patient comes in with their heart pounding, upset from that breakup or mad as hell at their mother, I give them a TIPP.

How to do it?

T is change your Temperature. Have you heard of the mammalian dive reflex? Try leaning over a sink or surface and placing cold water, ice, or a cold pack over the temples, eyes, and upper nose region for 30 seconds. This dive-like stance triggers a reflex that occurs in nature when mammals submerge in cold water. Think back to the last time you dove into a cold pool at the start of summer; you may recall the sensation of slowly cutting through the water with your arms, and a feeling of slowed time as you drifted up towards the surface. As we dive face-first into cold water, our heart rate slows and our breathing regulates as the body prepares to conserve energy for survival. We have engaged our parasympathetic nervous system and experience a calming effect. So next time you feel highly activated, distressed, upset, or angry, think "T for temperature" and try running cold water on your forearms, taking a hot or cold shower, chewing on ice, or just holding an ice cube in your hand. When we briefly change our temperature, we ground ourselves in the present moment and refocus.

I stands for Intense exercise. Intense exercise or brief bursts of exercise can be helpful in the grounding process. Intense exercise could be running around the house, lifting the knees up high, doing jumping jacks, or anything that increases the heart rate to the maximal amount. Think of this process as "using up" some of the energy that may be fueling high-energy emotions such as anger or anxiety. When in a low-energy state (e.g., feeling down, depressed, lethargic), getting the heart rate up will invigorate you.

P is Paced breathing. Paced breathing is exhaling longer than inhaling (I suggest five seconds in and seven seconds out). Paced breathing allows us to activate our parasympathetic nervous system as we regulate and slow our breath. With paced breathing, we breathe deeply into our lungs and diaphragm. As we slow the pace of our in breaths and out breaths, we may achieve five or six thoughtful breaths per minute. Some people refer to deep breathing as "having a pill in your pocket." In other words, breathing is a highly accessible skill—available to you at all times no matter where you are—and one that can be very effective in calming and steadying you when emotion is running high.

P is Progressive muscle relaxation. This exercise combines breathing and visualization to help you release tension and anxiety. If you do this with your child, one of you might be the "guide" while the other performs the exercise; then switch. Or you can try it together once you have gone through the visualization process a few times. The text here is written to appeal to a young child, although visualizing can be fun and funny at any age. Feel free to embellish or replace my images with your own! You can say the script below, which I often record so children can do it on their own before bed:

First, begin with a relaxing breathing pattern. [You can pick one described above if you'd like: alternate nostril, square, or paced.]

Next, we will relax each part of the body in turn.

Begin with the hands. Pretend you have a whole tangerine in your hands. Now squeeze it hard. Try to squeeze all the juice out. Feel the tightness in your hands and arms as you squeeze. Now drop the tangerine. Compare how your muscles feel when they tight and when they are relaxed.

Let's move to the arms and shoulders.

Pretend you are a furry, lazy cat. You want to stretch. Stretch your arms out in front of you. Raise them up high over your head. Way back. Feel the pull in your shoulders. Stretch higher. Now just let your arms drop back to your side.

Okay, kitty, let's stretch again. Stretch your arms out in front of you. Raise them over your head. Pull them back, way back. Pull hard. Now let them drop quickly. Notice how your shoulders feel more relaxed.

This time, try to touch the ceiling. Stretch your arms way out in front of you. Raise them way up high over your head. Push them way, way back. Notice the tension and pull in your arms and shoulders. Hold tight now. Then let them drop very quickly and feel how good it is to be relaxed. It feels good and warm and lazy.

Here comes a pesky old bee. He lands on your nose. Try to get him off without using your hands. That's right, wrinkle up your nose. Make as many wrinkles in your nose as you can. Scrunch your nose up real hard. Good. You've chased him away. Now you can relax your nose.

Oops, that bee is back. Right back in the middle of your nose. Wrinkle up your nose again. Shoo him off. Wrinkle it up hard. Hold it just as tight as you can. Shoo bee. Shoo! Phew, he flew away. You can relax your face.

Notice that when you scrunch up your nose, your cheeks and your mouth and your forehead and your eyes all help you, and they get tight too. So, when you relax your nose, your whole body relaxes too, and that feels good. Uh-oh. This time that bee has come back, but this time he's on your forehead. Make lots of wrinkles. Try to catch him between all those wrinkles. Hold it tight now.

Okay, you can let go. He's gone for good. Now you can just relax. Let your face go smooth, no wrinkles anywhere. Your face feels nice and smooth and relaxed.

Hey! Here comes a cute baby rhino. But he's not watching where he's going. He doesn't see you lying in the grass, and he's about to step on your stomach. Don't move. You don't have time to get out of the way. Just get ready for him. Make your stomach very hard. Tighten up your stomach muscles real tight. Hold it. It looks like he is going the other way. You can relax now. Let your stomach go soft. Let it be as relaxed as you can. That feels so much better.

Oops, he's coming this way again. Get ready. Tighten up your stomach. If he steps on you when your stomach is hard, it won't hurt.

Make your stomach into a rock. Okay, he's moving away again. You can relax now. Settle down, get comfortable, and relax. Notice the difference between a tight stomach and a relaxed one. That's how we want to feel–nice and loose and relaxed.

This time imagine that you want to squeeze through a narrow fence and the boards have nails on them. You'll have to make yourself very skinny if you're going to make it through. Suck your stomach in. Try to squeeze it up against your backbone. Try to be skinny as you can. Then relax. Feel your stomach being warm and loose.

Okay, let's try to get through that fence again. Squeeze up your stomach. Make it touch your backbone. Get it real small and tight. Get it as skinny as you can. Hold tight. You've got to squeeze through. Okay, you got through that narrow little fence! You can relax now. Settle back and let your stomach come back out where it belongs.

You can feel good now.

Now pretend you are a ballerina and need to point those toes. Point them hard and straight. You'll probably need your legs to help you get your leg stiff and your toes pointed. Relax your feet. Let your toes go loose and feel how nice it feels to be relaxed.

This time you want to push your toes up and keep them stiff and try to grab them with your hands, stretching and grabbing as hard as you can. Let your leg muscles help push your feet towards you and stretch as much as you can. Okay. Come back out now. Relax your feet, relax your legs, relax your toes. It feels so good to be relaxed. No tenseness anywhere. You feel kind of warm and tingly.

Stay as relaxed as you can. Let your whole body go limp and feel all your muscles relaxed. Go from stiff as a robot to loose as a rag doll.

Let's do another deep breath in and count to 10.

In a few minutes, I will ask you to open your eyes, and that will be the end of this practice session. As you go through the day, remember how good it feels to be relaxed. Sometimes you need to make yourself tighter before you can be relaxed, just as we did in these exercises. Practice these exercises every day to get more and more relaxed. Practice, and you can do our exercises and nobody will know.

Today is a good day, and you are ready to feel very relaxed. You've worked hard and it feels good to work hard. Very slowly now, open your eyes and wiggle your muscles around a little. Very good. You've done a good job. You're going to be a super relaxer.

TIPP SKILLS are amazing during the holidays when children may be so excited by the idea of presents and family parties but then do not sleep well. For example, if my youngest daughter gets jealous of her older sister's new gifts (my older daughter gets more mature toys), this often creates issues between them. I will ask her to splash some cold water on her face in the bathroom and practice breathing exercises (hold her breath, breathe in for five seconds and out for seven). This is both Temperature and Paced breathing (the T and P of TIPP), which are both great coping skills.

Intense exercise is such a powerful tool for damping down emotions. I tell patients to sprint around their house. Patients feel so much better after they get their heart rate up. Exercise works by releasing feel-good endorphins, preventing muscle atrophy, and helping promote restful sleep and prevent insomnia.

Progressive muscle relaxation is magic for those excited, sleepless nights before Santa comes or the Hanukkah gifts arrive. I love the Calm app, which has great programs for kids. Or I sit them both on their beds and then go through the progressive muscle relaxation script described above. I had my friend record the script in his funniest British accent. The kids adore it and always beg me to put it on. Teens may prefer more advanced scripts than the one given above, but everyone will enjoy being soothed to sleep with a calm voice and seemingly simple exercises. My nine-year-old especially loves becoming a furry, lazy cat and sttrreeeccchiinnggg, often meowing and purring when we get to that part.

TIPP skills are a great way to use simple techniques taught by psychologists to cope with intense emotions. Parents and children, try them out together. You will not be disappointed!

RAIN to control emotions
• • • •

Teenagers are notoriously bad at controlling their emotions. And until their frontal lobes fully develop, it can be hard to dampen down the intensity (even some adults struggle with this). One technique that has been amazingly helpful with my patients comes from Michele McDonald, a senior mindfulness teacher, and is written about in Tara Brach's book *True Refuge*. Brach is a psychologist and expert in mindfulness. Using her expertise in Buddhist principles, she talks about a technique called RAIN.

RAIN means:

Recognize what is happening;

Allow the experience to be there, just as it is;

Investigate with interest and care;

Nurture it with self-compassion.

Brach advocates for Recognizing your emotion, whether it be anxiety, anger, fear, or confusion. Feel it in your body. For example, is your chest tightening, your stomach doing flips, your heart beating faster? Then allow all of that to happen. Personally, in place of Allow, I prefer to "Accept" the emotion; it may be unpleasant, but accepting it means not fighting against it. After that, you can Investigate the emotion. It is how we think about a negative event that usually makes the negative emotions persist. And finally Nurture, which I prefer to think of as "Non-attachment": our emotions, and our thoughts about our emotions, don't define who we are. Think of emotion as just the top of the wave, where in the bottom is who you really are—still and calm. Brach writes of emotions: "waves on the surface belong to your experience, but cannot injure or alter the measureless depth and vastness of your being." I couldn't agree more strongly, and I recommend following her work on Twitter and other platforms!

Emotion wrangling tricks

● ● ● ●

Core values are the beliefs we hold about ourselves, our present circumstances, and our future. Dr. Aaron Beck, the founder of CBT (cognitive behavioral therapy), argued that these core beliefs, which are usually formed during early childhood, become the way we see the world around us. In 2014 Beck Institute workshop, Dr. Beck explained that "unhealthy core beliefs are robust and will prevail in neutral situations such as when you fail at Ping-Pong and you feel bad afterwards, but a healthy person may have the same beliefs but not as robust, and can shrug off [the lost game] quickly."

Some core values are healthy and positive, such as a belief that "I am smart and capable," "Helping others is rewarding," or "Honesty makes me feel good." Core values that are negative–such as "I need to be perfect to be loved"–can create anxiety or lead to animotophobia (a fear of expressing one's emotions).

Children filter their experiences through the core values they have adopted. When faced with hardships–such as a breakup or an issue with a close friend–an individual with a healthy set of core values may be hurt but will approach their feelings in a reasonable way. They will know that life will go on, that they will form new relationships, and they will remind themselves of the strong relationships that they still have. Unhealthy core values, though, can lead to maladaptive assumptions: "This breakup means that I'm worthless," "I'll never fall in love," "No one likes me."

Teens with unhealthy core beliefs can sometimes undergo serious injury to their self-esteem. I have seen patients punish themselves, cut themselves, or, even worse, try to kill themselves after events that should be weathered as a normal part of social life. In terms of how it relates to sex, a healthy self-esteem is essential to a sex-positive life. When a teen comes into my office with low self-esteem, they are at risk for unsafe sexual behavior. Also, when they are having sex, they often cannot experience much pleasure as they are too inhibited. This often stems from their unhealthy core beliefs in which they find themselves undeserving.

Parents can be directly involved in the creation of healthy core beliefs, although this requires an assessment of their own core beliefs. Parents must ask *themselves* how they interpret events and respond to challenges before they can fully understand why their children respond as they do. Once maladaptive beliefs and assumptions are challenged on a personal level, this questioning can be extended to their children.

A child-friendly list of cognitive distortions

Cognitive distortions are types of distorted thoughts, often negative, that can illuminate unhealthy core beliefs. These types of cognitive distortions, originally coined by Dr. Beck, were later expanded upon by Dr. David Burns in his bestseller *Feeling Good: The New Mood Therapy*. As mentioned in chapter 1, you can think of a cognitive distortion as a thought hole: distorted, non-reality-based, illogical thinking. Below are descriptions of some of the nuances within the thought hole experience.

Negative filtering: Only paying attention to negative thoughts or information ("glass half empty"). Like the dot of ink that colors the entire glass of water. Only seeing the craters on the beautiful blue moon.

Discounting positive: Not paying attention to positive things or failing to consider positive events as important (scoring a 99 on the test and focusing on the 1 point that was missed).

Catastrophizing: Imagining the worst possible outcome ("If I fail this test, then I will fail the semester, do poorly in high school, and never make it to college.")

Fortune-telling: Predicting the future negatively ("I will fail this test, so what is the point in studying?").

Emotional reasoning: Confusing feelings with facts, and letting emotions shape your view of reality ("I am sad, so I have no friends").

Personalizing: Blaming yourself for everything even if the fault is with others, or there is no fault that should be assigned.

Blaming: Blaming someone else for something you did.

Mind reading: Assuming that you know the content of other people's thoughts. Although mind reading can happen in positive directions ("He really loves me") as well as negative ones ("That girl thinks I'm ugly"), many teenagers focus on the negative ("Those other kids are laughing at *me*").

Labeling: Deciding the worst about someone or yourself based on very little information. ("That person wears glasses, so they are a nerd").

Black-and-white thinking: Viewing situations or people in "all or nothing" ways ("I am rejected by everyone").

Regret: Focusing on what you could have or should have done differently in the past rather than what is possible now.

Unfair comparison: Always finding yourself lacking when you compare yourself with others.

Thought log exercise

Rational thought can be honed with training, just as one can train for other types of human activity. A thought log is like a diary where you can help your child evaluate their thoughts, and whether their thoughts are positive or negative. It is a regular exercise that can be used at any age, beginning as early as age seven.

Learning how to identify negative thought patterns is a skill that is not taught in schools, or even in most homes, but it is one that will benefit your child for their entire lifetime. One way to learn about thought patterns is by writing them down. Writing down the thoughts allows your child or teenager to identify distortions in their thinking and to shift their patterns. This is an essential part of what we call "mindfulness."

Mindfulness requires evaluating your thoughts in the present moment and deciding whether a thought is helping you or creating pain. Being able to step back and evaluate our thoughts is a gift, allowing us to develop rational and balanced responses to events.

There are now mobile applications that allow for thought logs, if you prefer using your phone, but make sure that the chart looks similar to what I have provided in the next few pages so that these categories are included.

On page 240 you will find an example of the thought log of a younger child (aged 7-10). Parents attempting to work on thought logs with children of this age might consider using a reward system, or filling out the chart together.

On page 241 is an example of the thought log of an older child, aged 10-13; and on page 242 is an example of the thought log of a teen, aged 13-17.

These examples can help you think about how to reevaluate your thoughts, and your child's, in order to be more rational and balanced. One's thoughts do not need to be grandiose, but should simply provide an alternate interpretation that one can work with to improve the future.

The double standard technique

Pretend that you are listening to a friend, not talking with yourself. Would you be kinder towards your friend than you are towards yourself in your internal dialogue?

Criticism and self-evaluation can be rational without being deflating. If your child says something like, "I always fail at tests," for example, you can help them rephrase their analysis to be more rational and balanced. Saying, "Sometimes I fail, but other times I do well on tests" would be a more accurate and healthy observation. Rational evaluations of one's appearance, abilities, social standing, or performance will not be framed in black-or-white terms, but rather in shades of gray.

Another technique is to ask your child to brainstorm other possible explanations for an event. If a friend has not returned a call, for example, it is possible that they are angry. But it also might be possible that they had family obligations that kept them from the phone, or that they were not feeling well, or that they were busy with homework.

Sample thought log of a child aged 7–10

Event	Thought	Emotion: 1–10	Cognitive distortion? If so, what type?	Rational thought	Emotion: 1–10
Johnny kicked the back of my chair.	Why does he hate me?	Sadness: 7 Frustration: 6	Mind reading	Maybe he is just having a bad day. He is likely not thinking about me at all. He did sit next to me at lunch, so it's possible this is not about me.	Sadness: 6 Frustration: 5
The teacher told me I got the answer wrong.	I am so stupid.	Shame: 7 Sadness: 5	Labeling	Everyone gets things wrong sometimes. I answered some questions correctly yesterday.	Shame: 5 Sadness: 3
Mom told me I can't play with Jack, because she doesn't have time to drive me.	Why is she so unfair? She is always so busy.	Anger: 6	Black-and-white thinking Emotional reasoning	She did drive me to Jack's last weekend. She told me she was sorry and she would make it up to me.	Anger: 5
My sister got to have the first pancake.	She is so annoying. Why does she always get to be first? Why am I always made to wait? She's my parent's favorite.	Anger: 8	Labeling Emotional reasoning	I did get the first cookie yesterday. My mom did take me shopping, just her and me yesterday.	Anger: 6

Sample thought log of a child aged 10–13

Event	Thought	Emotion: 1–10	Cognitive distortion? If so, what type?	Rational thought	Emotion: 1–10
Lucy wouldn't let me sit with her at lunch today; she told me the seat was taken.	I am such a loser.	Sadness: 8 Self-loathing: 7	Labeling	She was mean to other kids in the past. Jamie stood up for me. Why would I let what Lucy thinks of me define how I feel about myself?	Sadness: 7 Self-loathing: 5
Joe told me I was "retarded" in science lab.	He must totally hate me. I am so stupid. Why can't I just be normal?	Sadness: 8 Self-loathing: 5	Labeling	Joe is the kid in the class with the worst grades. I don't need to listen to him.	Sadness: 5 Self-loathing: 2
Brianna didn't text me back after I told her about my sprained ankle.	She totally doesn't care about me. She must think I am totally lame.	Shame: 6	Mind reading Labeling	She might be busy with her family. Why would she think I'm lame? We are best friends.	Shame: 5
No one complimented me on my new shirt.	Why doesn't my mother buy me nicer clothes? Why can't I be popular?	Frustration: 8	Blaming Labeling	Just because no one noticed my shirt doesn't mean my clothes are not nice. I have a good sense of style. Most days I am complimented.	Frustration: 6

Sample thought log of a teen aged 13-17

Event	Thought	Emotion: 1-10	Cognitive distortion? If so, what type?	Rational thought	Emotion: 1-10
No one has asked me to the prom yet.	I will be the only one there without a date. What's wrong with me?	Frustration: 9 Shame: 4	Fortune-telling Labeling	Prom is still three weeks away, and lots of people are just going with friends. It doesn't mean I am not worthy.	Frustration: 5 Shame: 2
I tried to speak to John and he didn't respond.	I will never have a boyfriend. I might as well give up.	Sadness: 8 Frustration: 6	Fortune-telling Black-and-white thinking	The fact that one guy is not responding does not mean that I will never have a boyfriend. I need to be patient.	Sadness: 7 Frustration: 5
Pam and Lucy went to the movies on Friday and didn't invite me.	Why would they do this to me? Maybe I am not cool enough to hang out with them. I am losing all my friends.	Frustration: 8 Shame: 5 Sadness: 6	Mind reading Fortune-telling	We don't all need to do everything together. We can all do things on our own.	Frustration: 5 Shame: 4 Sadness: 5
I was kissing John at the park, but then I had to sneeze.	He is going to think I am uncool. I am so awkward and weird.	Embarrassment: 6	Mind reading Fortune-telling	He probably didn't even notice. He may have been worried about himself.	Embarrassment: 5

Self-image exercise

Have your child write three words to describe themselves. Or, have them describe themselves from head to toe, beginning with their hair. You'd be surprised how many children, teens, or adults describe themselves negatively. When I ask my patients to go head to toe and describe themselves, it is shocking what I find they will say (even boys). It's always hard for me to fathom how the beautiful, healthy child in front of me can think so poorly of themselves and their body.

- ✕ Okay smile
- ✕ Crooked teeth
- ✕ Bent nose
- ✕ Bad skin
- ✕ Kinky hair
- ✕ A big mouth
- ✕ Small breasts
- ✕ Fat stomach
- ✕ Big arms
- ✕ Big thighs which don't touch
- ✕ Wide hips and fat legs
- ✕ Unattractive compared to my friends

I will grab a new sheet of paper (see next page), and ask them to incorporate new data into their distorted and rigid body image schema, rewriting each line as in the example below. I'll go through their answers with them, suggesting more positive and kinder ways to describe themselves.

Many teens blast their body as being unfit, for example, without realizing what a remarkable piece of engineering it is! Health can be taken for granted rather than being experienced as an amazing gift. When it comes to our self-image, we must learn to accept some things about who we are. We may be tall, short, muscular, or bony; some of these things can be changed through practices, such as working out,

- ✓ Nice smile
- ✓ White teeth
- ✓ Nose which allows me to smell delicious things
- ✓ Olive skin which protects me from the sun
- ✓ Curly hair
- ✓ Alluring lips
- ✓ Breasts which some day will provide nourishment for my children
- ✓ Healthy stomach which processes food without pain

- ✓ Muscular arms which allow me to play sports
- ✓ Strong muscular legs which allow me to dance
- ✓ Wide hips which my partner will find attractive and will allow me to bear children
- ✓ Body which allows me to run, dance, move, and do what I want to do without pain or illness

but others cannot. Learning to accept who we are, and to love the skin that we live in, is a pathway to happiness.

Learning to bend at the knees and accept the bad things life throws at us will also teach us to enjoy the good things. But learning is a process.

Owning your sexual story is the key to positive parenting

• • • •

Being able to talk about sensitive, taboo, or embarrassing topics requires you to come to terms with your own sexuality–your experiences, desires, fears, and values. Creating a dynamic and satisfying sexual story for both you and your child is thus another essential part of this journey. You can be the parent your child needs through sharing your own experiences and wisdom.

What is your "sexual story"?

It is not just your sexual history, although your sexual history is important in shaping that story. Your sexual story is also not determined by your relationships, although each relationship–whether with parents, friends, or lovers–has influenced it.

Your sexual story is the meaning that you make out of your past experiences and relationships and the way that you envision your future. Even someone whose life has been full of trauma or strife can take responsibility for creating a meaningful story out of those negative experiences that helps them live a fulfilling life.

Your sex life may evolve as you age, become a parent, or change partners. A dynamic sexual story helps you integrate these changes into your overall sense of who you are. As a parent, your own story definitely influences your child's developing story. It goes without saying that being a great role model is essential to sex-positive parenting. This requires reflecting on your memories, actions, emotional responses, and unconscious hopes and fears. When explored, this information can be used as a tool to teach and share knowledge with your children.

So, how do you own your sexual story?

Here are a few ways to reflect on your sexual story through exploring your personal narrative. Using techniques that come from cognitive behavioral therapy–a technique called cognitive reframing–you can spin that narrative not only to be more rational and balanced but so as to sift out the values you want to pass down. This exercise can be done through either writing or deep reflection.

Describing your situation as accurately as possible is the key to cognitive reframing: just like your child, your negative mind loves to see reality darker than it is, especially when something negative happens to you. Write your sexual story down from the first experiences of puberty to the great sexual encounters and painful ones. Try to remember to make sure you see reality as accurately as possible, including all the negatives and positives, without judgment (aka stating "that guy was an asshole"). Just the facts.

Illuminate your personal power: Just as your mind loves to see reality darker than it is, it also loves to portray you as way less powerful than you really are. With cognitive reframing, you want to accurately understand your contribution to how things went. There are some things about your sexual story that were out of your control (such as in the case of sexual assault). Incorporate radical acceptance into the reframing of your sexual story:

"All the events of my past led up to now. This moment is perfect just as it is, and with all of these experiences I can be the parent my child needs as I have the experience and the wisdom to share with them."

• • • • • • • • • • • •

Brainstorm alternative views: You want to find better alternative views of what has happened to you. If there is trauma, or events where you might have made a different choice, seek a redemption narrative. The redemption narrative (frame) tells the story of a life where tough events also bring something good (with time), such as knowledge. Decide which pieces of your story you want to share and what is best kept confidential.

Why does unpacking your sexual story matter?

Knowing our own sexual stories is the key to being a great role model, and turning the cycle of intergenerational trauma into intergenerational wisdom. In addition, statistics show that parents who have

been sexually abused are more likely to have children who are sexually abused. This is a disturbing fact of intergenerational trauma.

How to get started

You can chart this out for yourself using the following template.

My sexual story

_____

_____

_____

My story with cognitive reframing

_____

_____

_____

. . . .

My family and what I know of their sexual story

_____

_____

_____

My family's story with cognitive reframing

_____

_____

_____

. . . .

Expression of affection and sexuality in my family

_____

_____

_____

How I wish to express affection and sexuality to my children

_____

_____

_____

. . . .

What my family and elders told me about sex

_____

_____

_____

What I wish they had told me

_____

_____

_____

. . . .

My early memories of sexual feelings and sexual play

_____

_____

_____

My early-memories story with cognitive reframing

_____

_____

_____

. . . .

My experiences with puberty

_____

_____

_____

My puberty story with cognitive reframing

_____

_____

_____

. . . .

The most positive sexual experience(s)

_____

_____

_____

My story with cognitive reframing

_____

_____

_____

. . . .

The most negative sexual experience(s)

_____

_____

_____

My story with cognitive reframing

_____

_____

_____

. . . .

**My sexual orientation and behavior from
the beginning until now: have there been changes?**

_____

_____

_____

My story with cognitive reframing

_____

_____

_____

. . . .

**History of risk-taking behaviors, including
STIs and unwanted pregnancies**

_____

_____

My story with cognitive reframing

_____

_____

_____

. . . .

Current sexual activity and preferences

_____

_____

_____

My story with cognitive reframing

_____

_____

_____

. . . .

What are my values around sex in terms of monogamy, honesty, fidelity?

_____

_____

My story with cognitive reframing

_____

_____

_____

. . . .

How I feel about my body

_____

_____

_____

My story with cognitive reframing

_____

_____

_____

. . . .

My child's birth story

_____

_____

_____

My story with cognitive reframing

_____

_____

_____

· · · · · · · · · ·

My fears for my child's sexual journey

_____

_____

_____

My hopes that I want to share

_____

_____

_____

What follows is a fictional example of how a parent could use this template to own their sexual story and pass down intergenerational wisdom.

My sexual story

My sexual story is filled with hard and bumpy times. My parents were not always happy and did not seem to have a great sex life. My first sexual experiences were unfulfilling. I was never open-minded regarding others and their sexualities when I was young. I learned to be more open as I got older and learned how to make myself experience sexual pleasure. That was liberating but took far too long.

My story with cognitive reframing (circle what to share with my child)

Learning about who you are sexually takes a long time and is a process. It's easy to get confused. You do not need to figure it out quickly. Trial and error helps you figure it out. As parents, we may make mistakes and may not always be the best role models. Feel free to ask us questions and I will try to be as open as possible. I want your journey to be fulfilling, and for painful times to be shared so we can all learn and grow together.

. . . .

My family and what I know of their sexual story

My mother never had a good sex life, as far as I can tell. She always had to cater to my father, who was strong and jealous most of the time. She never seemed free, always weighed down with obligation. My father had affairs, and I found this out and was very angry with the other women. It made me distrustful of others. I always blamed my father for cheating, yet I always wanted to be the center of attention, so I never confronted him. I was afraid he would reject me.

My family's story with cognitive reframing

My children should take ownership of their sexuality. If they are unhappy in a relationship, they should leave; obligations should never stand in the way of having fulfilling sex. But they can make demands and place boundaries. Those are good. I am NOT going to offer marriage and monogamy as the only way to live. I prefer promoting the ideals of honesty and integrity instead—those are the most important. And I will say: if the sex is not good and you love your partner, then work on it. There are so many modern-day tools available for people seeking to have a good relationship. Use them.

Expression of affection and sexuality in my family

My father was very affectionate and always hugging and kissing. My mother was often shut down. She never discussed feelings and love. I feel I can't touch or show love to my brother as he is older, he is very manly, and he gets so uncomfortable. As a result, we are not that close. I was discouraged from wearing sexy things, so I would hide my sexy outfits and makeup, and change after I left the house. I never had my boyfriends over and would have sex in the back seats of cars and at friends' houses.

My father would roughhouse with my brother, but never with me. I was allowed to kiss him and sit on his lap, but my brother was never allowed to do those things, or allowed to cry. He would say, "Ahh, stop crying!" I never saw my father cry except at a funeral for a child.

How I wish to express affection and sexuality to my children

My father was affectionate; I learned from him to love and to be kissed and caressed. Affection was very important to me growing up, which is why I love to touch and kiss you. I believe it's the foundation for great loving future relationships. I don't believe you should be one person at home and another outside your home. Your home is a safe place to be who you are and to dress how you want. As your parent, I will guide you on what I feel is appropriate in certain settings, but I want you to be YOU. I also want you to bring your partners over to the house and feel free to express appropriate affection and sexuality in our home. My home is your home; you shouldn't have to sneak around and hide things from me because you are afraid I won't accept you. I accept you—and if your behavior is inappropriate, I will tell you, and tell you why I think so, but I will do my best to not only accept your burgeoning sexuality but help it grow and flourish, so you have a loving and fulfilling series of relationships.

What my family and elders told me about sex

Nothing much. Use a condom . . . My mother told me once that if I got pregnant, she would take me to get an abortion. She did take me to the ob-gyn when I was of age, and paid for my birth control, but we never discussed what it was for. She never knew when I had my first sexual experience. It was never discussed. My father said things like, "Don't put up with shit from anyone," but that was it.

What I wish they had told me

I wish my parents had told me the importance of pleasure, how sex is intoxicating and exciting. I wish they had told me about yeast infections. I found that one out the hard way!

For my son and daughter: Please understand the importance of loving your partner in the moment, even if it is short-lived. Make sure to call them the next day, regardless of the circumstances. Never have sex for the first time with a new partner while intoxicated, and never leave a party drunk with a potential sex partner. Condoms break, and you can use six birth control pills the next day as a morning-after pill option. Waiting to have sex if you're not sure is a good idea.

For my daughter: Learn how to pleasure yourself first; orgasms don't often come from vaginal sex in most girls. I want you to be unafraid to show your partner how to please you; this is a good thing.

• • • • • • • • • •

My early memories of sexual feelings and sexual play

Masturbating in the shower with the shower head—not sure how young I was, but I remember doing it often. Playing boyfriend/girlfriend with a friend and kissing. Kissing my friend's labia on a dare and feeling horrible about it after; we never told anyone or discussed it again. I remember the feelings of watching Patrick Swayze in Dirty Dancing, *and the tingles when I saw the sex scene. I remember how good it felt kissing my girlfriend. Finding* The Joy of Sex *in my parents' closet and reading it cover to cover. Finding it fascinating.*

My early-memories story with cognitive reframing

Masturbation is normal and healthy. No one can pleasure you if you won't pleasure yourself. So do it as much as you would like. Figure out how to experience pleasure through all types of touch, such as having your hair brushed or your back scratched; this will help you figure out the way you want to be loved later.

Don't watch pornography before age 14. If you do see it, turn away. It will only make you more confused and won't help you feel good. I saw pornography by mistake, and regretted it. Look for good sources of information about sex. I read a book as a child that provided me with really great information. It was called *The Joy of Sex*, and I can even buy it for you to read if you like. I can also give you great information, or you can ask your auntie Michelle, or your counselor at school.

. . . .

My experiences with puberty

Puberty was hellacious. I hated myself. My breast development was quick; I had stretch marks. I couldn't figure out my body in space. I hated my first periods, which were heavy and painful. I didn't know about tampons; I had constant leaks. I never knew to take Motrin for pain. I wanted the boys to notice me, but they didn't, except to tease me. I wanted to have sex; the feeling was intense, so I looked to find whatever I could. I could not understand why I had to wait so long. I was so immature; I thought I knew more than I did. I did not understand why my body was changing so fast. I gained weight so fast; my feet were so big. I thought I wasn't cute like my friends. I worried about being popular all the time.

My puberty story with cognitive reframing

Puberty is hard. I hated growing up so fast. I worried about the changes in my body. Stretch marks are normal and will fade; I had them and I love my body now. Breasts will allow you to nurse a child. Menstrual cycles are a pain in the ass—can't sugarcoat it. But they allow you to carry a child—what a gift! The best thing that happened to me is you. I want to show you how to use tampons to deal with the bleeding. I will get you special Thinx period panties to avoid leaking. Use pain relievers to make periods better.

For my son: So what if you are smaller than the other boys? You will catch up. Hygiene is important: you must take showers every day. Please feel your testicles and if anything feels strange (like a raisin underneath the skin), tell me. Please use deodorant; I don't want to have to remind you. No one likes smelly aftershave. Masturbation is normal and healthy. Remember to leave tissues next to your bed so I don't have to change your sheets all the time. If you mess up the sheets, grab a new one and leave the messy one in the laundry room. Please ask me anything you want. Your penis will be perfect, I promise— more than enough for your partner! If you develop breast tissue, it will go away; it's not breasts, just puberty. Talk to me. I am not a boy, but I am experienced. I am not shy. There is time for everything, so don't rush, relish each experience from the first kiss onwards.

. . . .

The most positive sexual experience(s)

There are so many. When my friend gave me a vibrator in college, this was life-changing. I realized the role of clitoris in sex because of it. Realizing I could have multiple orgasms through my partner Matt. Having sex for days on end with my husband when we first met. Making sex tapes on an old video recorder.

My story with cognitive reframing

Positive sexual experiences come from knowing your own body and being able to relay that information to your partner. Sex toys for both masturbation and in sex with a partner can help you figure it out.

The key is being able to communicate in sex exactly what feels good, and this came with the openness of my partners in the past.

The most negative sexual experience(s)

Being trapped and almost raped several times, usually when drunk and separated from my friends, but one time, through no fault of my own, when lying in my dorm without the door locked.

My first husband didn't let me use sex toys. He thought he should be enough. He was offended if I asked to use them. Sex was boring; it resulted in the demise of our marriage.

My story with cognitive reframing

I was almost assaulted—thank God I was not hurt. I made some poor choices and left a party with someone I didn't know. I forgot to lock my dorm in college. Sexual assault can happen to anyone, but it is more likely to occur when you're drunk or high, so be aware of this at all times. Don't be afraid to walk out at any time for any reason. Don't leave your friends when they are drunk or high, for any reason. You don't need to do anything that doesn't feel good. Consent can be rescinded at any time for any reason. If you don't have chemistry, don't feel obligation. It is okay to walk away from a relationship even if you are committed, as your happiness should be a number one priority as long as you do it with honesty and take care of your obligations.

· · · · · · · · · ·

My sexual orientation and behavior from the beginning until now: have there been changes?

No, I always thought I was a little bisexual, but I wasn't sure completely. I decided to start dating men. I really like men. I did have a threesome once. I liked that. I like being with my second husband, he is good. I feel that I made a good choice.

My story with cognitive reframing

It's okay to experiment. You can be with all genders—you don't need to choose. It is better to be open and flexible until you find someone you want to be committed to. Even then, experimentation no matter what you want can be good as long as honesty and boundaries are clear ahead of time. You can tell me if you might be attracted to the same sex. I will love you no matter what, and I will be so proud you were brave enough to tell me.

. . . .

History of risk-taking behaviors, including STIs and unwanted pregnancies

I got pregnant in college, and I got an abortion. My boyfriend came with me, and my mom paid. I was too lazy to get my pill refilled. This was the price. It was stupid; I regret it, and I think about it often. I am remorseful; it could have been avoided, the procedure was pain-ful, and I was ashamed and still am. I am now using an IUD called Mirena. It's great. I wish I had known about the importance of birth control when I was 16.

My story with cognitive reframing

Our biology is not hard to figure out. Preventing pregnancy is easy, and I can help. Please come to me. IUDs are great; let's put one in as soon as you become sexually active. Please use condoms—I don't want you to get a disease. I will pay for your STI tests every year. I won't be angry if they come back positive, no matter what. I will help you navigate those waters.

For my son: Please be responsible. I will buy you many condoms. I will never let them run out; I will keep them in your room in end-less supply, and you can give them to your friends if they need some. Please discuss birth control with your partners, and encourage them to tell their parents. I am also happy to talk to your girlfriends—let's be collaborative. No sex when drinking, and please have sex in a safe place. Do not send naked photos as a teenager; you can go to jail. Never forward any naked pictures/videos of anyone, even if you did not take them; this is revenge porn, and it is really bad, and it's an act of violence that takes away consent.

Current sexual activity and preferences

Romance and sex life are good, not great; we have gotten into some monotony and routine. I learned from my first marriage that I need to work on this. Vacation sex is better.

My story with cognitive reframing

I didn't get it right the first time, which is why I got divorced. Your father and I need to work on our marriage to keep it spicy. Us having sex is good for you guys; it means that we can stay connected. It is good for the brain and for our relationship. Relationships take work.

· · · · · · · · · ·

What are my values around sex in terms of monogamy, honesty, fidelity?

Don't cheat; don't lie; talk about boundaries. When I got cheated on in my first marriage, it hurt really bad. When my father cheated, it hurt really bad. Trust is important, but forgiveness is also important. I am determined not to let my previous experiences color my current relationship.

My story with cognitive reframing

Do your best not to cheat or lie, but you don't have to share everything if it is going to hurt the other person. For example, you don't have to share every detail on every person you've ever slept with or everyone you have a crush on. You can love in the moment. Don't promise what you likely can't deliver. Fairy tales are for storybooks. Always call or reach out to the person after you have sex to tell them how wonderful they are even if you don't plan to have sex with them again. Being friends with your previous partner is mature.

· · · · · · · · · ·

How I feel about my body

I am overweight. I hate that. I sometimes catch myself talking about that in front of my children. It makes me feel bad. I hate the wrinkles above my eyebrows; I wish I could get plastic surgery to fix them. I want to have less cellulite; I wish I didn't have varicose veins. I take care of my body, try to eat right and groom as well as I can. I have great breath capacity. I love myself despite the above. It took some time to come to that conclusion.

I feel sexy a lot of the time. I like to dress sexy; I like to dance around and turn my husband on. He always notices me; he loves my breasts, and I love them too.

My story with cognitive reframing

My body is healthy. I don't have any health problems. I am so lucky. I can dance and move and swim. I can learn new sports. I focus on health instead of weight. Imperfections are part of who we are. We are sexy no matter what flaws we have. Sexy is also a state of mind. Confidence is sexy; curves are sexy. Men are sexy when they flatter women and make them feel good. We all need to take care of ourselves to be as sexy as we can!

. . . .

My child's birth story

I was older, and I didn't get pregnant the natural way. I needed help with IVF for my first pregnancy. It was tough to figure out how many eggs to implant. I felt guilty about the money. I was worried my whole pregnancy. I worked hard to have the baby without a C-section. The epidural was amazing. When she came out, I thought I was in heaven. For the second birth, I was more confident; I pushed him out and watched with a mirror. He was also amazing. They are very loved.

My story with cognitive reframing

We needed some help from technology to have my daughter. I will explain to both children that, in my daughter's case, a doctor took sperm from Dad and an egg from me and put them in a dish, and then that was put back inside me. I will tell my daughter: you grew in my uterus, and you were born after a lot of work and pushing. Dad was happy. You were very wanted. For my son—it was easier. I will tell them both that, in my son's case, we had sex and the sperm came out of Dad and into my vagina and into my uterus and fertilized an egg during my ovulation. You are both perfect just the way it happened. We are lucky.

. . . .

My fears for my child's sexual journey

That I will raise a daughter who hates herself, or who will get raped, or who will be in an unhappy marriage.

That my son will be a pervert, or a predator, or have bad manners.

That they will not love themselves, or they will not experience the pleasure I have. That they won't be able to commit and will be sex addicts.

That they won't give me grandchildren. I want grandchildren.

My hopes that I want to share

I want you both to have fulfilling sex lives. You can express your gender and sexual orientation in a way that makes you happy. I hope that your sexual journey won't result in distress or sadness or depression, that you will have pleasure and love, and that, hopefully, you will give me grandchildren.

11

OMG Guide: Fast Reference Q&A for Talking to Your Kids about Sex

• • • •

Q. At what age should I start talking about sex with my child?

. . . .

A. As soon as they can talk! Begin with the basics, such as naming body parts correctly (penis, vulva, vagina, anus). Tell them to let you know immediately if someone touches them on those parts besides parents/caregivers or a doctor. Studies show this understanding can actually cut down on sexual abuse and assault (see pages 34-35). And then, at about age five, fill them in about biology basics, such as sperm and egg creating a baby, which grows in the uterus. You can tell them the baby is created when the penis enters the vagina and sperm (seeds) are released, which then enters the uterus and fertilizes the egg, and forms the baby. This is called "sex" (see chapter 2). You'll fill in more details about intimacy, love, and pleasure when they are ready–around age nine.

Q. What is normal in terms of sexualized play as a child? What isn't normal and what do I need to watch out for?

. . . .

A. During the elementary years, children usually pair off and play mostly with their own gender. As this is an imaginative phase, children may act out scenes of a sexual nature, such as make their dolls kiss or go on dates, or mimic behaviors they observe in adults. Children may play "boyfriend" and "girlfriend" with each other, for example, or play-act with family roles (mother, father, baby). Making sure that your child understands and respects bodily boundaries will prevent such play from progressing too far. Signs that your child could have been sexually abused are: regression to previously outgrown behaviors, for example bed-wetting or thumb-sucking; abnormal sexual behaviors such as rubbing their genitals against the floor or other people in a sexualized manner; grabbing other children's or parents' genitals; or knowledge of advanced sexual language and behaviors in play with other children. (See more on pages 35-39.)

Q. At what age do most kids start masturbating, and what should I tell my child about it?

• • • •

A. Most kids start masturbating as toddlers, and little boys often get quick erections from it but don't begin ejaculating until puberty. Desires to masturbate or think about sex are normal. Masturbation should be ignored, and not commented on, but if it is happening often and in public, then remind them it's okay to touch their penis/vulva, and yes it feels good, but to please do it in private. Be clear that it is never okay to touch anyone else's penis or vulva. Also, if your child is at adolescence, talk about hygiene when masturbating (see pages 41-42).

Q. Is it okay for my child (even of the opposite sex) to see me naked?

• • • •

A. Yes, this is a great way for children to learn what adult bodies of all ages look like. It shows them that, yes, even Grandma/Grandpa or other older adults can get naked. This may also reduce fear of change during puberty and beyond. It is a great way to promote body-positive self-esteem. Of course, this comes with the caveat of keeping eroticism out of the picture. Consider family skinny-dipping (common in northern European cultures). See "8 things to know about nudity" (pages 54-56).

Q. How do I teach my child about boundaries?

• • • •

A. The idea of a "bubble" around the child's body may help them express their feelings if they do not want to be touched or if another child is acting aggressively towards them. Parents can model the use of a bubble if a child is pulling their hair or jewelry, kicking, or otherwise entering their space inappropriately, indicating with their hands, "This is my bubble, do not enter it." Also, give them permission to say no to unwanted touch no matter what type (see chapter 3).

Q. What can I do if my child walks in on me having sex?

• • • •

A. This is every parent's nightmare. Although it is normal for children to go through developmental stages where they engage in sexual exploration or flirtatious behavior, it is important for all adults and older siblings in the house to maintain appropriate boundaries. Children should never engage in or even watch family members engage in sexual behavior. Lock the bedroom door. Turn on loud music so that nothing can be heard outside the door. Lock your sex toys in a safe. But . . . what if your child accidentally walks in on you having sex? How you handle the situation, of course, will depend on the specific circumstances, the age of the child, and the relationship you have built up to that point.

Do not scream or get angry, or act ashamed; this is a normal thing and it's nothing to be ashamed about. Kids pick up immediately on your emotional reactions, and the weirder you act, the more fearful or "grossed out" they will be about sex. Ask them to leave the room, and then later, when you're dressed, do not lie to them (i.e., don't say you were wrestling or doing yoga), but rather tell them you were having sex, and this is what parents do who love each other (see pages 72-73).

Q. My child is being bullied based on their appearance/sexuality. What can I do?

· · · ·

A. If you suspect your child is being seriously bullied, try to reach out to the parent of the other child or to the school's psychological support services to intervene, as this can get very serious quickly. If it is not serious bullying and more like teasing, I think trying to normalize it is good, perhaps saying something like, "Everyone gets teased and the best thing to do is ignore it and focus on the people in your life who like and care about you."

For more information, see page 109.

Q. What do I do if my child questions their gender identity?

· · · ·

A. Children change their views on their identity many times, and it is normal for them to want to dress like the other sex or play with toys more common to the other gender. Allowing them to express their gender identity freely, within reason, will prevent gender dysphoria (feelings of sadness related to gender identity). If changing their gender becomes a more permanent preference, then get support (see pages 171-73) to help them navigate this complicated landscape.

Q. Should a father tell his daughter about sex?

· · · ·

A. YES! This is so important. Don't be afraid. Dads, you have a very important role to play. And doing so will help develop body-positive self-esteem, and prevent negative sexual outcomes. Opposite-sex role models should not simply be understood as examples of "male" or "female" behavior, but also as a way to combat cultural stereotypes. Adult men can model respect and empathy for young girls, showing that these are qualities for both men and women to display. If a young girl is exposed to a loving male figure, she will develop expectations for how men can treat women. This is a win-win, because even if the child doesn't pick the opposite sex as an intimate partner, they are still going to have to work and interact with the opposite sex in their day-to-day life, and should have high standards in ALL environments for how they are treated by the opposite sex. (See pages 170-71.)

And don't leave out the pleasure talk. It's even more important than the "Don't let anyone touch you whom you don't want" talk. It's crucial to add that if it doesn't feel good and it's not pleasurable, then don't do it; pleasure is the whole point of sex (see page pages 85-86).

Q. What do I do if my child is wearing something that I think is too sexually explicit for their age?

• • • •

A. It depends on the context. Let them express their individuality as long as it's not a question of something permanent (such as a tattoo or piercing). Encouraging appropriate clothing for school, or sports, is important. Explain that the focus there is on learning or achieving, not on looks, and therefore in those settings you may need them to change. For more on this topic, see pages 96-99.

Q. What is an appropriate age for my child to have sex?

• • • •

A: There is no exact age, as bodies and minds develop differently for each child. I think a child having sex before age 15 is always inappropriate, as their bodies and minds are likely too immature to handle the responsibility. Things you should make sure they understand are: who they want to have sex with and for what reasons, how their partner feels about it, having a great plan for contraception and knowing how to use it, knowing where and when they will have sex (hopefully, in your home or another very safe place), and understanding the emotional and physiological effects of sex. They should also understand peer pressure to have sex and ways to combat it, never to have sex when intoxicated, and STIs and how to prevent them. (See chapter 5.)

Q. What can I do to contribute to my teenager's sex-positive self-esteem?

. . . .

A. Explain media manipulation, such as airbrushing (show YouTube videos of how this works). Discuss and monitor your child's social media to make sure they are keeping it appropriate, and stress that most kids do not live the fabulous lives they might appear to have on social media. Praise the right traits in your kids, such as strength, intelligence, and kindness, rather than looks. Never talk about being thin, but rather stress healthy eating. MOST IMPORTANT: Never denigrate your body in front of your children. Be a good role model. (See pages 94-99.)

Q. Can younger children fall in love?

. . . .

A. I have seen children fall utterly and crazily "in love" with other children, speaking about them constantly, wanting to be with them, and jealously guarding them from other friendships. I have seen them absolutely heartbroken after the loss of a childhood friendship, to the point of serious depression and suicidal thoughts (even in a nine-year-old). For more on this topic, see pages 105-8.

Q. My child touched someone inappropriately. How do I respond?

. . . .

A. Don't panic. Many times this is a part of normal developmental play. Lack of education around boundaries is likely the reason. For more on this topic, see pages 36-37.

Q. What are the most important things to tell my teen about sex?

. . . .

A. Explain the emotional and physiological effects of sex, that consent must happen verbally and at every stage of initiation of a sex act, and that priority must be on your partner's pleasure. Don't be afraid of pillow talk!

Even if the relationship is not going to last forever, it's okay to love *in the moment*. (See more in chapter 5, especially page 139.)

Q. What do I tell my child about pornography?

. . . .

A. Most pornography is acting. Consent is obtained offscreen. If pornography is upsetting them, they shouldn't continue watching it. For more on this topic, see chapter 6.

Q. How do I introduce a new partner into my child's life?

. . . .

A. Do not bring your child into your dating life. When it is time to introduce a new partner to your child, plan a fun activity like ice skating or visiting the zoo where everyone can be involved. The time frame should be limited, allowing the child time to process afterwards. For more on this topic, see pages 219-20.

Q. What is the best way to impart wisdom about sex to my child?

. . . .

A. By owning your own sexual story and passing on intergenerational wisdom, not trauma. Parental disclosures about your own sex life should always be carefully considered, but they can be very useful. There is a great exercise for this in chapter 10 starting on page 244.

Conclusion

THE END... but it's just the beginning for you!

So many of the suggestions in this book are common sense, and you were probably already doing many of them before you read the book. I hope in reading it you feel reassured you are on the right track, certainly from the Shameless Psychiatrist's perspective! If you learn a few new tricks, and get to put them to use, then all the time I spent writing this book will have been worth it.

I do not talk about my family much in this book, as the focus of my experience comes from my work with patients. But I am trying to practice what I preach with my own young children. They are beautiful humans, and though I make mistakes all the time (especially when I'm struggling to strike a work-life balance or when I am tired or overwhelmed), they know about sex, and they love their bodies. They dance naked freely in their bedroom at night, playing a song called "Shake Your Booty." We have so much fun discussing body parts and the functions of each, and they are always fascinated by the marvels of the human mind and body. When I pick up *It's Not the Stork!* and try to read it to them AGAIN (sex talks must be ongoing), they take it out of my hand and explain to me all about the penis, vagina, eggs, sperm, etc., and how it all works. I love when I hear them educating their friends or correcting the misinformation other children might be passing on, laughing when they tell me that there are actually kids at school who think babies come out of the belly button.

Empowering them and all the other children in my practice has led me to write this book. I cannot do enough to change the way children are raised if I settle for only treating 30 patients a week in my practice. I needed to get this information out. And so I pass the torch to you, the parents reading this. You can change your own children and help influence the other parents in your sphere to do the same with theirs. Don't leave it up to the gym teacher at school, or the kid across the street who is four years older. This is your family's journey, and raising a sex-positive child is going to mean that someday your child will be very happy in life. I can't wait for you to test this out, as all the parents have done in my practice, and get back to me with incredible stories about your children's future experiences. So, my friends, go forth and multiply, and once you do, read this book on how to raise them right!

Acknowledgments

TO EXPRESS my thanks, I must start from the very beginning. My father told me I was going to be the surgeon general someday. Sorry, Dad, but I think you would still be proud. And to my mother, who is unflappable, despite her obvious discomfort at some of my content. Thanks for the proofreading and always being a supporter of whatever I do.

I would also like to thank my mentors at St. Vincent's and NYU, Drs. Matthew Pravetz, Harold Koplewicz, Roy Boorady, Xavier Castellanos, and Jess Shatkin.

From the beginning of this book, there was Laura Stokes-Greene, Amy Richardson, Guru and Green, and Cristina Cuomo. Thanks for never getting tired of my neediness and always pushing me to finish. And to Katherine Frank, who lent that bit of academia and wisdom. To Caitlin Fitzpatrick for her boots on the ground and whose help allowed me to be present with my patients. In the middle, there was the marvelous Jenny Diaz, who brought the spunk I needed to some dry times. Thanks for the name "Shameless Psychiatrist."

At the end there was Page Two. Can a publisher save a book? They saved mine. Thank you for your wisdom.

To Alexander, who was unwavering in his support and love. Thank you over and over to infinity.

Notes

Chapter 1: An Introduction to Shameless Psychiatry
• • • •

parent–adolescent communication plays a protective role: C. McNeely et al., "Mothers' Influence on the Timing of First Sex among 14- and 15-Year-Olds," *Journal of Adolescent Health* 31, no. 3 (2002): 256-65, DOI: 10.1016/s1054-139x(02)00350-6; K.S. Miller et al., "Patterns of Condom Use among Adolescents: The Impact of Mother-Adolescent Communication," *American Journal of Public Health* 88 (1998): 1542-44; L. Widman et al., "Parent-Adolescent Sexual Communication and Adolescent Safer Sex Behavior: A Meta-analysis," *JAMA Pediatrics* 170, no. 1 (2016): 52-61, DOI: 10.1001/jamapediatrics.2015.2731.

teens who have regular conversations with their parents: S.C. Martino et al., "Beyond the 'Big Talk': The Roles of Breadth and Repetition in Parent-Adolescent Communication about Sexual Topics," *Pediatrics* 121 (2008): e612-18, DOI: 10.1542/peds.2007-2156.

too few adolescents talk with *anyone* about sexual topics: Ibid.; J.A. Shoveller et al., "Socio-cultural Influences on Young People's Sexual Development," *Social Science and Medicine* 59, no. 3 (August 2004): 473-87, DOI: 10.1016/j.socscimed.2003.11.017.

1 in 10 children will be sexually abused before their 18th birthday: C. Townsend and A.A. Rheingold, "Estimating a Child Sexual Abuse Prevalence Rate for Practitioners: A Review of Child Sexual Abuse Prevalence Studies," Darkness to Light, 2013, D2L.org/1in10.

1 in 7 girls and 1 in 25 boys will be sexually abused before they turn 18: Ibid.

44 percent of rapes with penetration occur to children under age 18: *National Crime Victimization Survey*, 2002, Bureau of Justice Statistics. Statistic calculated by staff at Crimes against Children Research Center.

Victims younger than 12 account for 15 percent of those raped, and another 29 percent of rape victims are between 12 and 17: L.A. Greenfeld, *Sex Offenses and Offenders: An Analysis of Data on Rape and Sexual Assault*, 1997, US Department of Justice, Bureau of Justice Statistics, NCJ-163392, bjs.gov/content/pub/pdf/SOO.PDF.

"ten thousand hours": Malcolm Gladwell, *Outliers: The Story of Success* (New York: Little, Brown, 2008).

documentary about Ruth Bader Ginsberg: Betsy West and Julie Cohen, directors, *RBG* (Magnolia Pictures, Participant Media, and CNN Films, 2018).

need for all parents to have rights protected, regardless of gender: *Weinberger v. Wiesenfeld* 420 U.S. 636 (1975) was a decision by the US Supreme Court that unanimously held that the gender-based distinction under 42 U.S.C. § 402(g) of the Social Security Act of 1935—which permitted widows but not widowers to collect special benefits while caring for minor children—violated the right to equal protection secured by the Due Process Clause of the Fifth Amendment to the US Constitution.

same-sex partners could do just as good a job as opposite-sex partners: H.M. Bos et al., "Same-Sex and Different-Sex Parent Households and Child Health Outcomes: Findings from the National Survey of Children's Health," *Journal of Developmental and Behavioral Pediatrics* 37, no. 3 (2016): 179-87, DOI: 10.1097/DBP.0000000000000288.

by some measures, same sex-parents can do even better: N.K. Gartrell, H.M. Bos, and N.G. Goldberg, "Adolescents of the U.S. National Longitudinal Lesbian Family Study: Sexual Orientation, Sexual Behavior, and Sexual Risk Exposure," *Archives of Sexual Behavior* 40, no. 6 (2011): 1199-1209, DOI: 10.1007/s10508-010-9692-2; N. Gartrell, H. Bos, and A. Koh, "National Longitudinal Lesbian Family Study: Mental Health of Adult Offspring," *New England Journal of Medicine* 379, no. 3 (2018): 297-99, DOI: 10.1056/NEJMc1804810; D. Mazrekaj, K. De Witte, and

S. Cabus, "School Outcomes of Children Raised by Same-Sex Couples: Evidence from Administrative Panel Data," 2018, semanticscholar.org/paper/School-Outcomes-of-Children-Raised-by-Same-Sex-from-MAZ-REKAJ-Witte/d5f9246adc36732e8d7c26f230202ce977d1191c. Please see also the National Longitudinal Lesbian Family Study, which is the longest-running prospective investigation of lesbian mothers and their children. This organization has produced many studies to support the claim that same-sex parents are as capable as heteronormative parents. See their website at nllfs.org for more information.

CBT has proven valuable for troubled families: Child Welfare Information Gateway, *Alternatives for Families: A Cognitive-Behavioral Therapy (AF-CBT)* (Washington, DC: US Department of Health and Human Services, Children's Bureau, 2013), childwelfare.gov/pubPDFs/cognitive.pdf; K. Thirlwall et al., "Treatment of Child Anxiety Disorders via Guided Parent-Delivered Cognitive-Behavioural Therapy: Randomised Controlled Trial," *British Journal of Psychiatry* 203, no. 6 (2013): 436-44, DOI: 10.1192/bjp.bp.113.126698.

CBT for treating anxiety and depression in children: J.S. March et al., "The Treatment for Adolescents with Depression Study (TADS): Long-Term Effectiveness and Safety Outcomes," *Archives of General Psychiatry* 64, no. 10 (2007): 1132-43, DOI: 10.1001/archpsyc.64.10.1132.

CBT for reducing behavioral problems: D.G. Sukhodolsky et al., "Behavioral Interventions for Anger, Irritability, and Aggression in Children and Adolescents," *Journal of Child and Adolescent Psychopharmacology* 26, no. 1 (2016): 58-64, DOI: 10.1089/cap.2015.0120.

CBT for raising self-esteem and academic performance: P. Waite, F. McManus, and R. Shafran, "Cognitive Behavior Therapy for Low Self-Esteem: A Preliminary Randomized Controlled Trial in a Primary Care Setting," *Journal of Behavior Therapy and Experimental Psychiatry* 43 (2012): 1049-57, DOI: 10.1016/j.jbtep.2012.04.006.

CBT for preventing substance use: D. Deas and S.E. Thomas, "An Overview of Controlled Studies of Adolescent Substance Abuse Treatment," *American Journal on Addictions* 10, no. 2 (2001): 178-89, DOI: 10.1080/10550490 1750227822.

CBT for improving mental health in teens: Graham J. Emslie et al., "Treatment of Resistant Depression in Adolescents (TORDIA): Week 24 Outcomes," *American Journal of Psychiatry* 167, no. 7 (2010): 782-91, DOI: 10.1176/appi.ajp.2010.09040552; L.D. Seligman and T.H. Ollendick, "Cognitive-Behavioral Therapy for Anxiety Disorders in Youth," *Child and Adolescent Psychiatric Clinics of North America* 20, no. 2 (2011): 217-38, DOI: 10.1016/j.chc.2011.01.003.

Dr. Marsha Linehan and DBT: Marsha Linehan, *DBT Skills Training Manual*, 2nd ed. (New York: Guilford Press, 2014).

progress teens make in DBT groups: Ibid.

authoritative parenting is characterized by high levels of emotional warmth, support, and responsiveness: A.E. Guyer et al., "Temperament and Parenting Styles in Early Childhood Differentially Influence Neural Response to Peer Evaluation in Adolescence," *Journal of Abnormal Child Psychology* 43, no. 5 (2015): 863-74, DOI: 10.1007/s10802-015-9973-2.

authoritarian parenting: Ibid.

"forbidden toy" experiment: J.L. Freedman, "Long-Term Behavioral Effects of Cognitive Dissonance," *Journal of Experimental Social Psychology* 1, no. 2 (1965): 145-55, DOI: 10.1016/0022-1031(65)90042-9.

effects of parenting style on children: A.E. Guyer, J.S. Silk, and E.E. Nelson, "The Neurobiology of the Emotional Adolescent: From the Inside Out," *Neuroscience & Biobehavioral Reviews* 70 (2016): 74-85, DOI: 10.1016/j.neubiorev.2016.07.037; A.E. Guyer et al., "Temperament and Parenting Styles."

adolescents with authoritarian parents: J.R. Bun et al., "Effects of Parental Authoritarianism and Authoritativeness on Self-Esteem," *Personality and Social Psychology Bulletin* 14, no. 2 (1988): 271-82, DOI: 10.1177/0146167288142006; T.C. Rothrauff et al., "Remembered Parenting Styles and Adjustment in Middle and Late Adulthood," *Journal of Gerontology Series B: Psychological Sciences and Social Science* 64 (2009): 137-46, DOI: 10.1093/geronb/gbn008; M. Uji et al., "The Impact of Authoritative, Authoritarian, and Permissive Parenting Styles on Children's Later Mental Health in Japan: Focusing on Parent and Child Gender," *Journal of Child and Family Studies* 23, no. 2 (2014): 293-302, DOI: 10.1007/s10826-013-9740-3.

negative, high-conflict parenting: I. Sandler et al., "Effects of Father and Mother Parenting on Children's Mental Health in High and Low Conflict Divorces," *Family Court Review* 46 (2008): 282-96, DOI: 10.1111/j.1744-1617.2008.00201.x.

negative parenting and higher levels of sexual activity: M.A. Longmore et al., "Parenting and Adolescents' Sexual Initiation," *Journal of Marriage and Family* 71, no. 4 (2009): 969-82, DOI: 10.1111/j.1741-3737.2009.00647.x.

Bobo doll study: A. Bandura, D. Ross, and S.A. Ross, "Transmission of Aggression through Imitation of Aggressive Models," *Journal of Abnormal and Social Psychology* 63 (1961): 575-82, DOI: 10.1037/h0045925.

children watch and imitate their parents: S. Duman and G. Margolin, "Parents' Aggressive Influences and Children's Aggressive Problem Solutions with Peers," *Journal of Clinical Child & Adolescent Psychology* 36, no. 1 (2007): 42-55, DOI: 10.1080/15374410709336567.

women with childhood experiences of physical abuse or aggression: E.K. Chung et al., "Parenting Attitudes and Infant Spanking: The Influence of Childhood Experiences," *Pediatrics* 124, no. 2 (2009): e278-86, DOI: 10.1542/peds.2008-3247.

positive parenting techniques: S.M. Eyberg and E.A. Robinson, "Parent-Child Interaction Training: Effects on Family Functioning," *Journal of Clinical Child Psychology* 11, no. 2 (1982): 130-37, DOI: 10.1080/1537 4418209533076; S.C. Kennedy et al., "Does Parent-Child Interaction Therapy Reduce Future Physical Abuse? A Meta-analysis," *Research on Social Work Practice* 26, no. 2 (2016): 147-56, DOI: 10.1177/104973151 4543024.

Chapter 2: Teaching about Bodies through the Stages

• • • •

sex offenders of children avoid children who know names of body parts: M. Elliott, K. Browne, and J. Kilcoyne, "Child Sexual Abuse Prevention: What Offenders Tell Us," *Child Abuse & Neglect* 19, no. 5 (1995): 579-94, DOI: 10.1016/0145-2134(95)00017-3; M.C. Kenny et al., "Child Sexual Abuse: From Prevention to Self Protection," *Child Abuse Review* 17 (2008): 36-54, DOI: 10.1002/car.1012.

A Patient's Story: Names and identifying details of all patient and personal stories in this book have been changed to protect the anonymity of those I work with.

children who touch others inappropriately: See "If Your Child May Be Harming Another Child," RAINN, rainn.org/articles/if-your-child-may-be-harming-another-child.

your child says someone else touched them inappropriately: See "National Resources for Sexual Assault Survivors and their Loved Ones," RAINN, rainn.org/national-resources-sexual-assault-survivors-and-their-loved-ones.

in Amsterdam it is all about the dos: Bonnie J. Rough, *Beyond Birds & Bees: Bringing Home a New Message to Our Kids about Sex, Love, and Equality* (New York: Seal Press, 2018).

HPV vaccine: Centers for Disease Control and Prevention, "Recommendations on the Use of Quadrivalent Human Papillomavirus Vaccine in Males–Advisory Committee on Immunization Practices (ACIP), 2011," *Mortality and Morbidity Weekly Report* 60, no. 50 (2011): 1705-8, ncbi.nlm.nih.gov/pubmed/22189893.

CDC and pediatricians recommend 11- and 12-year-olds receive HPV vaccine: Centers for Disease Control and Prevention, "FDA Licensure of Bivalent Human Papillomavirus Vaccine (HPV2, Cervarix) for Use in Females and Updated HPV Vaccination Recommendations from the Advisory Committee on Immunization Practices (ACIP)," *Mortality and Morbidity Weekly Report* 59, no. 20 (2010): 626-29, ncbi.nlm.nih.gov/pubmed/20508593.

recent studies suggested nonsexual transmission of HPV: E.J. Ryndock and C. Meyers, "A Risk for Non-sexual Transmission of Human Papillomavirus?" *Expert Review of Anti-infective Therapy* 12, no. 10 (2014): 1165-70, DOI: 10.1586/14787210.2014.959497.

girls' earlier introduction to sexual activity linked to depression: H. Gonçalves et al., "Age of Sexual Initiation and Depression in Adolescents: Data from the 1993 Pelotas (Brazil) Birth Cohort," *Journal of Affective Disorders* 221 (2017): 259-66, DOI: 10.1016/j.jad.2017.06.033.

earlier introduction to sexual activity and alcohol use, multiple sexual partners, and STIs: P.A. Cavazos-Rehg et al., "Number of Sexual

Partners and Associations with Initiation and Intensity of Substance Use," *AIDS and Behavior* 15, no. 4 (2011): 869-74, DOI: 10.1007/s10461-010-9669-0.

pain during sex: D. Herbenick et al., "Pain Experienced during Vaginal and Anal Intercourse with Other-Sex Partners: Findings from a Nationally Representative Probability Study in the United States," *Journal of Sexual Medicine* 12, no. 4 (2015): 1040-51, DOI: 10.1111/jsm.12841.

Chapter 4: Happy Humans! Helping Kids Form Healthy Relationships for Life

• • • •

happiness comes from forming stable relationships: R.J. Waldinger et al., "Security of Attachment to Spouses in Late Life: Concurrent and Prospective Links with Cognitive and Emotional Wellbeing," *Clinical Psychological Science* 3, no. 4 (2015): 516-29, DOI: 10.1177/2167702614541261.

Harvard's landmark study of adult development: George Eman Vaillant, *Aging Well: Surprising Guideposts to a Happier Life from the Landmark Harvard Study of Adult Development* (Carlton North, Australia: Scribe, 2006).

happiness correlated to forming intimate relationships: M. Ardelt, K. Gerlach, and G. Vaillant, "Early and Midlife Predictors of Wisdom and Subjective Well-Being in Old Age," *Journals of Gerontology: Series B* 73, no. 8 (2018): 1514-25, DOI: 10.1093/geronb/gby017.

Berkeley happiness project: Vaillant, *Aging Well.*

"blue zones," geographic regions where people live the longest: D. Buettner and S. Skemp, "Blue Zones: Lessons from the World's Longest Lived," *American Journal of Lifestyle Medicine* 10, 5 (2016): 318-21, DOI: 10.1177/1559827616637066.

"The Power 9": You can also find it on Buettner's blog: bluezones.com/2016/11/power-9.

the need to "downshift": Dan Buettner, *The Blue Zones of Happiness: Lessons from the World's Happiest People* (Washington, DC: National Geographic Society, 2017).

Okinawan Confucian mantra: Ibid.

"Plant Slant": Ibid.

push fiber on your girls: M.S. Farvid et al., "Dietary Fiber Intake in Young Adults and Breast Cancer Risk," *Pediatrics* 137, no. 3 (2016), DOI: 10.1542/peds.2015-1226.

one of his categories is "Belong": Buettner, *The Blue Zones*.

"The social networks of long-lived people . . .": Ibid.

both male and female adolescents more likely to have discussions about sex with mothers: C. Diiorio et al., "Communication about Sexual Issues: Mothers, Fathers, and Friends," *Journal of Adolescent Health* 24, no. 3 (1999); 181-89, DOI: 10.1016/S1054-139X(98)00115-3.

Canadian prime minister Justin Trudeau and feminism: Justin Trudeau, "Why I'm Raising My Kids to Be Feminists," *Marie Claire*, October 11, 2017, marieclaire.com/politics/a12811748/-trudeau-raising-kids-feminist.

6 tips for assertive communication: These ideas were taken with three sources in mind: Marsha Linehan, DBT *Skills Training Handouts and Worksheets*, 2nd ed. (New York: Guilford Press, 2015), 47-49; David D. Burns, *When Panic Attacks: The New, Drug-Free Anxiety Therapy That Can Change Your Life* (New York: Morgan Road Books, 2006), 305; and Matthew McKay, Jeffrey C. Woods, and Jeffrey Brantley, *The Dialectical Behavior Therapy Skills Workbook: Practical DBT Exercises for Learning Mindfulness, Emotion Regulation & Distress Tolerance*, 2nd ed. (Oakland, CA: New Harbinger, 2019), see, especially, the chapters on interpersonal relationships.

Dr. David Burns talks about anger: David D. Burns, *Feeling Good: The New Mood Therapy* (repr., New York: Harper, 2008).

positive self-esteem reduces adolescents' likelihood of engaging in risky sexual behaviors: J.L. Kerpelman et al., "Engagement in Risky Sexual Behavior: Adolescents' Perceptions of Self and the Parent-Child Relationship Matter," *Youth & Society* 48, no. 1 (2016): 101-25, DOI: 10.1177/0044118X13479614.

in a study, 56 normal-weight college women were exposed to sexually objectifying music videos: I.H. Mischner et al., "Thinking Big: The Effect of Sexually Objectifying Music Videos on Bodily Self-Perception in Young Women," *Body Image* 10, no. 1 (2013): 26-34, DOI: 10.1016/j.bodyim.2012.08.004.

not how much time overall was spent on Facebook that had a negative effect: E.P. Meier and J. Gray, "Facebook Photo Activity Associated with Body Image Disturbance in Adolescent Girls," *Cyberpsychology, Behavior, and Social Networking* 17, no. 4 (2014): 199-206, DOI: 10.1089/cyber.2013.0305.

Facebook can actually extend social support: L.A.S. Shapiro and G. Margolin, "Growing Up Wired: Social Networking Sites and Adolescent Psychosocial Development," *Clinical Child and Family Psychology Review* 17, no. 1 (2014): 1-18, DOI: 10.1007/s10567-013-0135-1.

person cannot feel anger and joy simultaneously: Burns, *Feeling Good*.

youth who are incessantly teased or bullied: M. M. Bucchianeri et al., "Multiple Types of Harassment: Associations with Emotional Well-Being and Unhealthy Behaviors in Adolescents," *Journal of Adolescent Health* 54, no. 6 (2014): 724-29, DOI: 10.1016/j.jadohealth.2013.10.205.

Tamera's Parents' School: Check out their website for more information at tamera.org/parents-school.

Chapter 5: Sexual Initiation

• • • •

age of sexual debut has gone up: L.B. Finer and J.M. Philbin, "Sexual Initiation, Contraceptive Use, and Pregnancy among Young Adolescents," *Pediatrics* 131, no. 5 (2013): 886-91, DOI: 10.1542/peds.2012-3495.

when parents express care for their kids there is a delay in sexual initiation: M.A. Longmore, W.D. Manning, and P.C. Giordano, "Preadolescent Parenting Strategies and Teens' Dating and Sexual Initiation: A Longitudinal Analysis," *Journal of Marriage and Family* 63 (2001): 322-35, DOI: 10.1111/j.1741-3737.2001.00322.x.

over-monitoring can result in backlash: M.A. Longmore et al., "Parenting and Adolescents' Sexual Initiation," *Journal of Marriage and Family* 71, no. 4 (2009): 969-82, DOI: 10.1111/j.1741-3737.2009.00647.x.

teen pregnancy rate has dropped to a third of what it was in 1990: Guttmacher Institute, "Adolescent Sexual and Reproductive Health in the United States," fact sheet, September 2019, guttmacher.org/fact-sheet/american-teens-sexual-and-reproductive-health. In 2013, the adolescent pregnancy rate reached a record low of 43 pregnancies per 1,000 women aged 15 to 19, indicating that fewer than 5 percent of females in this age group became pregnant. This rate represented a decline to just over a third of the peak rate of 118 per 1,000, which occurred in 1990. See also K. Kost, I. Maddow-Zimet, and A. Arpaia, *Pregnancies, Births and Abortions among Adolescents and Young Women in the United States, 2013: National and State Trends by Age, Race and Ethnicity* (New York: Guttmacher Institute, 2017), guttmacher.org/report/us-adolescent-pregnancy-trends-2013.

how we are entering into a sex recession: Kate Julian, "Why Are Young People Having So Little Sex?" *Atlantic*, December 2018, theatlantic.com/magazine/archive/2018/12/the-sex-recession/573949.

Adults too are having sex less frequently: NORC's General Social Survey, norc.org/Research/Projects/Pages/general-social-survey.aspx.

4 steps to flirting: David D. Burns, *When Panic Attacks: The New, Drug-Free Anxiety Therapy That Can Change Your Life* (New York: Morgan Road Books, 2006).

fear will always be there to greet us: Brené Brown, *The Power of Vulnerability: Teachings of Authenticity, Connection, and Courage*, audiobook (Louisville, CO: Sounds True, 2013).

Dr. Albert Ellis challenged himself to speak to 100 women: Kristen Tobias, "A Bronx Tale," The Albert Ellis Institute, February 20, 2015, albertellis.org/bronx-tale.

Jason Silva talks about rejection: Jason Silva, "Have You Ever Been Rejected?," Instagram video, 3:47, instagram.com/tv/B2kEDaTlW-c/?igshid=jmypnzt3adyu.

rejection is good practice for what will happen all the time in life: Burns, *When Panic Attacks*.

risk taking offers neurological rewards: Frances E. Jensen with Amy Ellis Nutt, *The Teenage Brain: A Neuroscientist's Survival Guide to Raising Adolescents and Young Adults* (New York: HarperCollins, 2014).

adolescents generally try to avoid this discussion: Jess Shatkin, *Born to Be Wild: Why Teens Take Risks, and How We Can Help Keep Them Safe* (New York: Penguin, 2017), 188.

the underlying biological processes that occur when we become intimate with someone: S.W. Kim et al., "Neurobiology of Sexual Desire," *NeuroQuantology* 11, no. 2 (2013): 332-59, DOI: 10.14704/nq.2013.11.2.662; C.S. Carter, "The Role of Oxytocin and Vasopressin in Attachment," *Psychodynamic Psychiatry* 45, no. 4 (2017): 499-517, DOI: 10.1521/pdps.2017.45.4.499; B.P. Acevedo et al., "Neural Correlates of Long-Term Intense Romantic Love," *Social Cognitive and Affective Neuroscience* 7, no. 2 (2012): 145-59, DOI: 10.1093/scan/nsq092.

dopamine levels in the brain increase during adolescence: Shatkin, *Born to Be Wild*, 47.

teens who have earlier sexual initiation more likely to have depression: D.D. Hallfors et al., "Adolescent Depression and Suicide Risk: Association with Sex and Drug Behavior," *American Journal of Preventive Medicine* 27, no. 3 (2004): 224-31, DOI: 10.1016/j.amepre.2004.06.001.

teens girls who engage in oral sex less satisfied in relationships: G.V. Holway and K.H. Tillman, "Timing of Sexual Initiation and Relationship Satisfaction in Young Adult Marital and Cohabiting Unions," *Journal of Family Issues* 38, no. 12 (2017): 1675-1700, DOI: 10.1177/0192513X15613826.

Teen Vogue featured an article addressing anal sex: Gigi Engle, "Anal Sex: Safety, How Tos, Tips, and More," *Teen Vogue*, November 12, 2019, teenvogue.com/story/anal-sex-what-you-need-to-know.

Chapter 6: Annihilating the Risks

• • • •

On average, 8- to 12-year-olds use just under five hours' worth of screen media per day: Pew Research Center, "Teens, Social Media & Technology 2018," May 2018, pewresearch.org/internet/2018/05/31/teens-social-media-technology-2018; V. Rideout and M.B. Robb, *The Common Sense Census: Media Use by Tweens and Teens, 2019* (San Francisco: Common Sense Media, 2019), commonsensemedia.org/sites/default/files/uploads/research/2019-census-8-to-18-key-findings-updated.pdf.

Michelle Carter pressured her boyfriend to kill himself via a string of text messages: Ray Sanchez and Natisha Lance, "Judge Finds Michelle

Carter Guilty of Manslaughter in Texting Suicide Case," CNN, June 17, 2017, cnn.com/2017/06/16/us/michelle-carter-texting-case/index.html.

"cyberbullicide": S. Hinduja and J.W. Patchin, "Bullying, Cyberbullying, and Suicide," *Archives of Suicide Research* 14, no. 3 (2010): 206-21, DOI: 10.1080/13811118.2010.494133.

Dr. Sameer Hinduja and Dr. Justin Patchin reported results: S. Hinduja and J.W. Patchin, "High-Tech Cruelty," *Educational Leadership* 68, no. 5 (2011): 48-52, researchgate.net/publication/286965892_High-Tech_Cruelty.

one great study found that 93 percent of boys and 62 percent of girls viewed pornography: S. Chiara, J. Wolak, and D. Finkelhor, "Rapid Communication: The Nature and Dynamics of Internet Pornography Exposure for Youth," *Cyberpsychology & Behavior* 11, no. 6 (2008): 691-93, DOI: 10.1089/cpb.2007.0179.

only 12 percent of parents are aware of what their kids are watching: Covenant Eyes, *Pornography Statistics: 250+ Facts, Quotes, and Statistics about Pornography Use,* 2015 edition (Owosso, MI: Covenant Eyes, 2015), covenanteyes.com/lemonade/wp-content/uploads/2013/02/2015-porn-stats-covenant-eyes.pdf.

they aren't just watching missionary sex scenes: Maggie Jones, "What Teenagers Are Learning from Online Porn," *New York Times Magazine,* February 7, 2018, nytimes.com/2018/02/07/magazine/teenagers-learning-online-porn-literacy-sex-education.html.

one soon-to-be-published study by Dr. Debby Herbenick and Dr. Bryant Paul: As part of the survey, led by Dr. Herbenick, a professor at the Indiana University School of Public Health and director of the university's Center for Sexual Health Promotion, along with her colleague Dr. Paul, 614 teenagers aged 14 to 18 reported their experiences with porn.

not every porn viewer wants to act out what they have seen: E. Martellozzo et al., "'I Wasn't Sure It Was Normal to Watch It...': A Quantitative and Qualitative Examination of the Impact of Online Pornography on the Values, Attitudes, Beliefs and Behaviours of Children and Young People," NSPCC and Children's Commissioner for England (London: Middlesex University, 2016), DOI: 10.6084/m9.figshare.3382393.

2016 meta-analysis of pornography research: P.J. Valkenburg, "Adolescents and Pornography: A Review of 20 Years of Research," *Journal of Sex Research* 53, no. 4-5 (2016): 509-31, DOI: 10.1080/00224499 .2016.1143441.

excessive porn watching creating a supernormal stimuli: D.L. Hilton, "Pornography Addiction: A Supranormal Stimulus Considered in the Context of Neuroplasticity," *Socioaffective Neuroscience of Psychology* 3 (2013): 20767, DOI: 10.3402/snp.v3i0.20767.

Tinbergen created artificial bird eggs: Nikolaas Tinbergen, *The Study of Instinct* (Oxford: Clarendon Press, 1989).

supernormal stimuli activate our natural reward system: Frederick Toates, *How Sexual Desire Works: The Enigmatic Urge* (Cambridge: Cambridge University Press, 2014); T. Love et al., "Neuroscience of Internet Pornography Addiction: A Review and Update," *Behavioral Sciences* 5, no. 3 (2015): 388-433, DOI:10.3390/bs5030388.

watching porn can make you want novel stimulation: See TED Talk and online information by Gary Wilson, "The Great Porn Experiment," fightthenewdrug.org/media/video-tedx-talk-the-great-porn-experiment.

88.2% of porn videos contained physical aggression: A.J. Bridges et al., "Aggression and Sexual Behavior in Best-Selling Pornography Videos: A Content Analysis Update," *Violence against Women* 16, no. 10 (2010): 1065-85, DOI: 10.1177/1077801210382866.

The messages that porn disseminates about women: Gail Dines, *Pornland: How Porn Has Hijacked Our Sexuality* (Boston: Beacon Press, 2010).

you can liken the porn industry to a predatory capitalist industry: Interview with Dr. Gail Dines, "The Birds and the Bees—and Porn—in the Internet Age," NPR's *On Point*, June 17, 2019, wbur.org/onpoint/2019/06/17/children-porn-sexual-education.

teens who sext more likely to be sexually active: S. Madigan et al., "Prevalence of Multiple Forms of Sexting Behavior among Youth: A Systematic Review and Meta-analysis," *JAMA Pediatrics* 172, no. 4 (2018): 327-35, DOI: 10.1001/jamapediatrics.2017.5314.

sexting investigation in Virginia: "Police Hope Parents, Teens Will Learn from Sexting Case," *Richmond Times-Dispatch*, April 9, 2014,

richmond.com/police-hope-parents-teens-will-learn-from-sexting-case/
article_74707a13-6355-5842-a51f-8fd64bcb0dc2.html.

Jordan Johnson overdosed at a party home: Pei-Sze Cheng, "I-Team: Teen's
Drug Overdose at Notorious Party Home in Hamptons Captured on Snapchat, No Arrest," NBC New York, February 16, 2017, nbcnewyork.com/
news/local/party-drug-alcohol-overdose-east-hampton-long-island-
police-investigation-teen/393960.

Chapter 7: Teaching Radical Inclusion for Gender, Sexual, & Family Identities and Expressions

• • • •

**recent study by the CDC, 88 percent of high school students iden-
tified as heterosexual:** Centers for Disease Control and Prevention,
"Sexual Identity, Sex of Sexual Contacts, and Health-Related Behaviors
among Students in Grades 9-12–United States and Selected Sites, 2015,"
Mortality and Morbidity Weekly Report 65, no. 9 (2016): 12-202, DOI:
10.15585/mmwr.ss6509a1.

**same-sex couples about five times more likely to raise adopted
children:** Abbie E. Goldberg, *Lesbian and Gay Parents and Their Children: Research on the Family Life Cycle* (Washington, DC: American
Psychological Association, 2010). Also see resources from the National
Longitudinal Lesbian Family Study at nllfs.org.

**comparisons of gay, lesbian, and heterosexual parents found few dif-
ferences:** Ibid.

same-sex couples more likely to share child care: Ibid.

resources about parenting adopted children: See the resources by the
Center for Adoption Support and Education at adoptionsupport.org/
education-resources/for-parents-families/free-resources-links.

issues that might come up with adopted children: R.H. Farr, S.L. Forssell,
and C.J. Patterson, "Parenting and Child Development in Adoptive Families: Does Parental Sexual Orientation Matter?" *Applied Developmental
Science* 14, no. 3 (2010): 164-78, DOI: 10.1080/10888691.2010.500958.

reactive attachment disorder: A rare condition that occurs when children are exposed to extreme neglect or abuse during their early years.
This severe trauma results in inability to form appropriate bonds with
caregivers, or development of inappropriate relationships (or no recognition of boundaries) with adults.

places where nontraditional families find support: glaad.org, adoption
council.org, soloparentsociety.com, and chosenfamilylawcenter.org.

Chapter 8: A Parent's Ongoing Sexual Story

• • • •

Dr. Elisabeth Sheff has studied polyamorous families: Elisabeth Sheff,
*The Polyamorists Next Door: Inside Multiple-Partner Relationships and
Families* (Lanham, MD: Rowman and Littlefield, 2015).

"Border Families" and the need for diversity and multiplicity: Maria
Pallotta-Chiarolli, *Border Sexualities, Border Families in Schools*, Curriculum, Cultures, and (Homo)Sexualities Series (Lanham, MD: Rowman
and Littlefield, 2010), 222.

Chapter 10: Boost & Embolden
Self-Esteem in Your Child

• • • •

present moment doesn't just leap into being: Matthew McKay, Jeffrey
C. Wood, and Jeffrey Brantley, *The Dialectical Behavior Therapy Skills
Workbook: Practical DBT Exercises for Learning Mindfulness, Interper-
sonal Effectiveness, Emotion Regulation, and Distress Tolerance* (Oakland,
CA: New Harbinger Publications, 2007).

research suggests positive impacts of meditation: M. McGee, "Meditation and Psychiatry," *Psychiatry (Edgmont)* 5, no. 1 (2008): 28-41, ncbi.nlm
.nih.gov/pmc/articles/PMC2719544.

meditation and anxiety: S. Evans et al., "Mindfulness-Based Cognitive
Therapy for Generalized Anxiety Disorder," *Journal of Anxiety Disorders*
22, no. 4 (2008): 716-21, DOI: 10.1016/j.janxdis.2007.07.005.

meditation and aggression: T. Toneatto and L. Nguyen, "Does Mindful-ness Meditation Improve Anxiety and Mood Symptoms? A Review of the Controlled Research," *Canadian Journal of Psychiatry* 52 (2007): 260-66, DOI: 10.1177/070674370705200409.

meditation and suicidality: J.M. Williams et al., "Mindfulness-Based Cognitive Therapy for Prevention of Recurrence of Suicidal Behav-ior," *Journal of Clinical Psychology* 62 (2006): 201-10, DOI: 10.1002/jclp.20223.

meditation and depression: A. Finucane and S.W. Mercer, "An Explor-atory Mixed Methods Study of the Acceptability and Effectiveness of Mindfulness-Based Cognitive Therapy for Patients with Active Depres-sion and Anxiety in Primary Care," BMC *Psychiatry* 6 (2006): 14, DOI: 10.1186/1471-244X-6-14.

TIPP skills: Marsha Linehan, DBT *Skills Training Manual*, 2nd ed. (New York: Guilford Press, 2014). Available separately: Marsha Linehan, DBT *Skills Training Handouts and Worksheets*, 2nd ed. (New York: Guilford Press, 2015).

technique called RAIN: Tara Brach, *True Refuge: Finding Peace and Free-dom in Your Own Awakened Heart* (New York: Bantam Books, 2013). You can find more about this technique in Brach's YouTube videos and on her website: tarabrach.com/rain.

Tara Brach writes of emotions: Brach, *True Refuge*.

unhealthy core beliefs are robust and will prevail in neutral situations: Dr. Aaron Beck, "Negative Core Beliefs in CBT," Beck Institute workshop (video, 1:10), 2014, beckinstitute.org/negative-core-beliefs-in-cbt.

cognitive distortions: Based on Dr. Aaron Beck's principles of cognitive behavioral therapy as described in David D. Burns, *Feeling Good: The New Mood Therapy* (New York: HarperCollins, 2008).

beautiful, healthy child thinks poorly of themselves: M.M. Bucchianeri et al., "Body Dissatisfaction from Adolescence to Young Adulthood: Findings from a 10-Year Longitudinal Study," *Body Image* 10, no. 1 (2013): 1-7, DOI: 10.1016/j.bodyim.2012.09.001.

parents who have been sexually abused more likely to have children who are sexually abused: J.L. Borelli et al., "Maternal and Child Sexual Abuse History: An Intergenerational Exploration of Children's Adjustment and Maternal Trauma-Reflective Functioning," *Frontiers in Psychology* 10 (2019): 1062, DOI: 10.3389/fpsyg.2019.01062.

Chapter 11: OMG Guide: Fast Reference Q&A for Talking to Your Kids about Sex
• • • •

my child touched someone inappropriately: See "If Your Child May Be Harming Another Child," RAINN, rainn.org/articles/if-your-child-may-be-harming-another-child.

About the Author

DR. LEA LIS is the Shameless Psychiatrist.

Dr. Lis is a medical doctor who is a double board-certified adult and child psychiatrist. She has been working with families since the beginning of her psychiatric career.

She is uniquely positioned to help parents and children face many mental health challenges and live healthy lives. She has developed expertise in working with modern families of all types during her training and residency at St. Vincent's Hospital and New York University; she has further honed her approach in her own private psychiatric practice, Mindful Kid.

Psychiatry and medicine has been Dr. Lis' calling since the age of 15 when she started volunteering at Hillside Hospital. She now has a thriving clinical practice where she sees adults and children with all types of mental health issues in Southampton, New York.

Dr. Lis writes a well-received column for *Psychology Today,* Thrive Global, and *The Purist*, and has appeared as an authority on parenting on ABC, CBS, and NBC. She has been featured in numerous media outlets such as the *Chicago Tribune*, the *Washington Post*, and in niche publications like *Good Housekeeping*, and *Psychiatric News*. She has been interviewed as a mental health expert on multiple podcasts.

Dr. Lis is active in the American Psychiatric Association, having served as a member of their National Ethics Committee and on the Board of Trustees. She served as assistant clinical professor of psychiatry at New York University Medical Center, and has presented numerous symposia and workshops at the annual APA meetings and at the meetings of the Institute of Psychiatric Services. Her academic publications have appeared in the *Journal of Psychiatric Practice* and *Academic Psychiatry*.